Trauma and Madness in Mental Health Services

Noël Hunter

Trauma and Madness in Mental Health Services

palgrave
macmillan

Noël Hunter
New York, NY, USA

ISBN 978-3-319-91751-1   ISBN 978-3-319-91752-8   (eBook)
https://doi.org/10.1007/978-3-319-91752-8

Library of Congress Control Number: 2018942900

Cover photo © Kirill Makarov / Alamy Stock Photo

Printed on acid-free paper

This Palgrave Macmillan imprint is published by the registered company Springer International Publishing AG part of Springer Nature.
The registered company address is: Gewerbestrasse 11, 6330 Cham, Switzerland

PREFACE

Every day the news is filled with stories of sexual assault, murder, poverty, pervasive systemic racism, children suffering at the hands of caregivers, suicide, and bullying, among many others. Loneliness has become an epidemic, with broken relationships increasingly becoming the norm. What happens to the children whose parents are too stressed to nurture or too haunted by their own pain to notice? How do people learn to connect when they have learned nothing but rejection and marginalization? Where do people who are suffering go for help and support?

The human body, and brain, is designed to acclimate to the environment in which it exists. When children grow up feeling unsafe, when experiences (such as abuse or social marginalization) overwhelm their ability to cope, they find ways to adapt. When these adaptations begin to become problems (i.e., being constantly ready to fight, shutting down, not trusting others, creating alternative realities, experiencing altered states of consciousness, etc.), such individuals often end up as psychiatric patients and diagnosed as mentally ill. In so doing, the adaptive nature of their distressing behaviors risks being disregarded and, instead, these phenomena may only be seen as a deficit with one's traumatic past dismissed or ignored altogether.

Those whose psyches have become torn apart (dissociated) to an extreme degree and whose lives are led by fear and anxiety due to difficult childhoods frequently find themselves depicted as caricatures in both entertainment and mental health services. When they are portrayed in the media, the public too often is given stories of violent, crazed individuals who either have a genetic disease over which they have no control and/or are some kind of sideshow oddity. People are captivated by the characters in Sybil, United States of Tara, Psycho, Fight Club, Mr. Robot, Black Swan, Split, Fatal Attraction, A Beautiful Mind, and others while wondering and debating as just how to classify and categorize them. Because, of course, these characters are a "them" who could never be "us".

My initial motivation for exploring this topic and conducting the interviews upon which much of this book is based was a personal one: before becoming a clinical psychologist, I was considered by some to be a seriously mentally ill patient. When I was a child, I witnessed many family members who were diagnosed, drugged, hospitalized, and otherwise "treated" by standard mental health services. I believed that they had real illnesses that explained their sometimes abusive and volatile behaviors. Much like the general public, I could not understand why someone would refuse to take their medications and feared having my own children one day lest I pass on my genetic faults. The fact that there was unfathomable abuse throughout my entire family, that coldness and greed superseded nurturance and love, and that emotional neglect was balanced only by an intrusive lack of boundaries seemed irrelevant. The messages put forth by the powers that be were strong: mental illness is a life-long biological disease over which one has little control and trauma is essentially background noise.

I did not begin to understand the falsehood of these beliefs until I, myself, became a user of mental health services. Within six months of seeking help after a lifetime of abuse and trauma, I had accrued eight different diagnoses, was put on five potent "medications" that made daily living unbearable, had my entire personhood challenged and altered, and became suicidal for the first time in my life. Initially, I eagerly sought out and was grateful to receive a diagnosis. Somehow my pain was finally recognized and I could say that it was real. I came to believe that the only reason I functioned was because of all the drugs I was taking and my luck at getting such knowledgeable expert professionals in my corner. I told my clinicians with varying levels of enthusiasm how helpful they were and thought I could not live without their guidance and support.

Eventually, however, I came to fear mental health professionals more than I did the screaming phantoms I saw each night and the vicious voices in my head. Not only were my experiences in the mental health system re-traumatizing, but they also critically altered my view of myself and the world. Further, the dynamics between me and several of the mental health professionals I encountered eerily mirrored those with my abusers, therein creating a renewed sense of powerlessness, defectiveness, and profound self-hatred. Yet, I simultaneously found myself grateful to them for making me feel this way. There are few things more terrifying than realizing that you cannot trust your own mind; others taking control of your mind is one of them.

It took a long time, and beginning my own studies before I started to question the way I was treated, stopped listening to the so-called experts, and started to finally heal. I learned to allow myself to be all the things I was encouraged NOT to be (oppositional, non-compliant, sensitive, independent) in order for me to begin becoming a fully functional human being who could genuinely enjoy life. I learned to face my past, challenge my fears, and dare to trust my instincts. Admittedly, I did not do this alone and was fortunate to have the support of a non-traditional mental health professional along the way. There is such great value to the therapeutic process when fear and authoritarianism are left outside the therapy room; when the process is based on respect, openness, and authenticity. Sadly, it seems that the more problems one has, the less likely this is to be the case.

As I delved further into my studies, I was increasingly shocked as I discovered the vast research that refutes much of what we assume to be true when it comes to mental health. I felt embarrassed by some of my behaviors under the guise of being mentally ill and the ways in which I adapted to the various labels I was given. Once I stopped identifying with my diagnoses (for me, an absolute necessity to ending my desire to die), I started to learn who "I", with all of my various parts, was and began to grow. As I met others who had similar experiences, I eventually came to realize that what I had been through was common and not the result of a couple of careless, cruel, or uninformed clinicians; it was the result of a fundamentally broken system that regularly hurts its most vulnerable.

So many people are hurting and so few feel that mental health services can provide them with the relationships and support they need to truly heal. We live in a world where empathy and compassion are commodities, and relationships are secondary to material gain; the current mental health paradigm is a reflection of this culture. The continued rising rates of chronic mental health disability in tandem with rising mental health spending in the United States and elsewhere appear to substantiate this sense of futility: certainly not for all, but for far too many.

The arguments presented here are not new and certainly not isolated to a few eccentric individuals such as myself. Most of what we assume to be true and the scientific discoveries that are so frequently splashed across the pages of our newspapers and internet homepages are most often nothing more than ideological assertions based on faith and selective findings rather than objective science. The ongoing philosophy that we, the public, are taking in at a rapid pace is one that tells us we are sick for being sad and shutting down when things get tough; that if we cannot deal with abuse or rape or chronic oppression in a way that avoids disturbing others, then there must be something wrong with us; if we are angry and scream because we are fed up with not being heard or being told that we are worthless or less than, this is a sign that we are defective as human beings; and that these beliefs somehow are based in medicine and can help us. I make no claims to be neutral—I find these notions not only to be lacking scientific validity, but they can be, and frequently are, incredibly dangerous.

Readers are encouraged to follow up with the 800+ cited resources that explore in far greater depth than this book has room for the individual topics laid out in the following pages. People who are looking for ideas for their own or a loved one's healing journey are advised to question, continue becoming informed, and make decisions based on what feels right—there is no one-size-fits-all solution. While I have strong beliefs, grounded in both science and personal experience, the strongest belief of all is how important it is to honor the subjectivity and wonderful variability in being human. No one should ever be in the position of power to determine how someone else should live or experience their life, and I certainly am not trying to be any exception to this.

Although my experiences have influenced my approach to both my clinical work and research, it is the resounding voices of others who have also been there that inspires and informs everything I think and do. This book is based on interviews I conducted as part of my doctoral research with individuals who identified with a diagnosis of DID and were in varying states of their own recovery process. They volunteered to participate in a long process and shared their stories in a most vulnerable way with a complete stranger. Their courage and resilience astonish me, and I feel fortunate to have learned as much as I have from them. I have done my best to include these participants in several steps leading to the development of both my completed doctoral thesis and this book, and to honor their voices as a group. Inevitably, individual stories or ideas may be lost in this broad effort, and, as with any type of research about another's subjective experience, my personal biases may override some aspects of their messages. I have gone to great lengths to avoid this, including working closely with a dedicated team of not-so-like-minded volunteers, my dissertation committee, and my doctoral mentor, to develop the themes and suggestions put forth throughout this book. But, no form of research is without bias (no matter how much some researchers might argue otherwise), and I personally find it to be important to acknowledge this impact.

The following pages are my attempt to convey the story of others in the best way I could. Our voices come together collectively to express shared experiences and a united goal of increasing healing opportunities for those desperately in need. The public health costs of continuing as we have are not sustainable or acceptable. It is time that more of these voices are heard and that change begins to occur. Our humanity depends on it.

New York, NY   Noël Hunter

ACKNOWLEDGMENTS

This book is the result not only of the grueling process of completing my doctoral studies but also my own circuitous journey through trauma, breakdown, and transformation. It is a challenge to a system of which I am a part but also a plea for people to listen to those of us who have been there. Trauma affects us all on many levels, and to face its confusing and painful aftermath is unbearable for many; for this, I am incredibly grateful to all those who were a part of the journey leading to this book in all the various roles they played.

First and foremost, I would like to express my utmost appreciation to the individuals who volunteered their stories and their time during the study upon which this book is based. They allowed me to enter their worlds, ever so briefly, and disclosed painful and difficult experiences with a profound enthusiasm and dedication to helping others. The trust in me to share their stories and the vulnerabilities that were displayed are not taken for granted. I can only hope that I have honored their words and experiences as best possible.

My dissertation committee, who supported and guided me throughout the process of collecting, analyzing, and grappling with much of the information presented throughout this book, has been instrumental. Danielle Knafo, my advisor, defender, advocate, challenger, and ally, unfailingly supported and guided me throughout my schooling and after even when doing so may have threatened to prematurely age her by several years. Her attempts to tame my outspoken and politically incorrect manner have largely been unsuccessful, yet she continued to stand by me and believe in me nonetheless. Additionally, Andrew Moskowitz offered me wisdom, patience, and openness even when in fierce disagreement. And, my thanks also goes to Susanne Phillips, for her genuine kindness, constructive criticism, and insights.

A great deal of gratitude goes towards those who so generously offered their time and expertise reviewing early drafts of specific chapters. I want to thank Jay Joseph and Mike Jones for their sometimes awe-inspiring knowledge of the genetics and twin study research in psychiatry, and the heart with which they continue to stand against the status quo. I also want to thank Kimberly Glazier for her time, insights, collaboration, support, and ongoing friendship. Further, my appreciation goes to Leah Harris, a fierce advocate, leader, and inspiration to me and many others. Lastly, to Fran Grossman for her support, encouragement, and wisdom.

Thank you, also, to Breukelen Coffee House for essentially serving as my office for the past year. Anyone who lives in New York City knows the incredible fortune of finding a spot to spend endless hours with free Wi-Fi and room to work all for the price of a coffee. Plus, these folks are just awesome.

And, of course, I would be nowhere without my colleagues, friends, mentors, and teachers both in life and in formal education guiding me, believing in me, and challenging me to be honest, open, and reflective. Some of my darkest moments during this process were brought to light through their support, provocation, and wisdom. To just name a few, Tristan Barsky, Robert Keisner, Kateri Berasi, Debra Japko, Deb Chu, Melissa Shroeder, Peter Stastny, Eva Chiriboga, Eva Feindler, and Deborah Lawrence.

Lastly, I want to acknowledge all the men and women out there who are suffering and in need of help, but feel they have nowhere to turn. The state of the current mental health system is abysmal, and too many find themselves in the same harmful and oppressive dynamics that led them to ail in the first place. There are many working to change that, several of whom collaborated on this project. Please know that you are not alone.

CONTENTS

LIST OF TABLES

PART I

The Status Quo

CHAPTER 1

Introduction: Containing Multitudes

[Mental health treatment] was so re-traumatizing. It was so similar to the original trauma; people who do things to you and deny that they did it. They deny that they had any responsibility and put it all back on you and just, it reinforces how evil you must be for that to happen. P13

While the news and other media outlets regularly report advancements in mental health treatment and discoveries, rates of diagnosable mental illness have increased across the globe, disability rates have skyrocketed, and advocacy movements led by ex-patients and dissident mental health professionals have grown. Suicide is now the second leading cause of death among individuals aged 15–34 years (Centers for Disease Control and Prevention (CDC), 2013/2011), and almost a quarter of individuals who suicide were on antidepressants at the time of death (Parks, Johnson, McDaniel, & Gladden, 2010). Perhaps more disturbingly, recent evidence has demonstrated that as contact with psychiatric intervention increases, so too does completed suicide, suggesting the possibility that the current mental health system may be creating the very problems it purports to aid, at least for some (Hjorthoj, Madsen, Agerbo, & Nordentoft, 2014; Large & Ryan, 2014). And, although suicide rates and disability due to mental health continue to rise, so too does spending on traditional mental health care (e.g., Druss, 2006). Are we continuing to funnel money into a fundamentally broken system? Is it possible that the biomedical paradigm under which all of mental health care operates is actually creating circumstances that are making people worse? Evidence from across cultures appears to point in this direction.[1]

© The Author(s) 2018
N. Hunter, *Trauma and Madness in Mental Health Services*,
https://doi.org/10.1007/978-3-319-91752-8_1

Although the public is led to believe in the foregone conclusion that what is called mental illness is biological and genetic in nature and that medical advancements have led to new discoveries and improved treatments, this is not actually so certain. In fact, much of the scientific literature tends to dispute these assertions while instead demonstrating the extensive effects that adversity has on biology and overall mental health (Chap. 6). Adverse experiences, particularly in childhood (such as physical and sexual abuse, parental separation, bullying, parental death, foster care, neighborhood violence, poverty, racism, etc.), have been demonstrated to have a direct and dose-response relationship (meaning the more adversity, the greater the risk) with adult mental health issues like hearing voices, suicidality, drug abuse, experiencing altered states of consciousness, extreme and intense emotions, fragmented sense of self, obesity, depression, paranoia, beliefs in conflict with consensus reality, anxiety, and more (see, e.g., Bentall, Wickham, Shevlin, & Varese, 2012; Felitti et al., 1998; Janssen et al., 2004; Read, van Os, Morrison, & Ross, 2005). There is also some evidence indicating specificity, wherein certain adverse experiences appear to be related to specific psychic phenomena. For instance, being bullied as a child is closely related to intense paranoia, while sexual abuse is more closely related to hearing voices (Bentall et al., 2012). Yet, most research and treatment continues to focus on individual internal defects (i.e., "illness") that exist separate from one's developmental context or life circumstances, and a search for the ever-elusive genetic basis for these purported defects.

In 1980, posttraumatic stress disorder (PTSD) was included in the *Diagnostic and Statistical Manual of Mental Disorders* (*DSM-III*; American Psychiatric Association, 1980) as a diagnosis that recognized the traumatic nature of one very specific way that some express their emotional distress, namely, by experiencing flashbacks directly and obviously related to an original traumatic event, excessive arousal and alertness, fear, and avoiding reminders of the trauma. This inclusion was largely the result of political efforts on the part of American veterans of war, as opposed to the discovery of a new disease that exists in nature. During this period, women also increasingly had political power and a voice in the greater public discourse, and brought to public awareness the common experiences of childhood sexual abuse, rape, and domestic violence. This was the first time since that of Pierre Janet, in the late nineteenth century, and the early works of Sigmund Freud that the impact of trauma was recognized on a broad level (Chap. 2).

Since then, the field of trauma studies has continued to expand and the findings consistently support instinctual wisdom: people go mad, become aggressive, and are fearful because they have been profoundly hurt. Despite these findings, the biomedical paradigm continues to reign, treatment continues to be centered on a coercive and paternalistic framework, and "mental illness" is still asserted by many to be a real disease that is based in genetics and brain dysfunction. The trauma field at times perpetuates this both by separating out disorders based in trauma from what is believed to be more genetically determined illness, and by implying that trauma causes brain dysfunction that is permanent. Yet, brain difference does not equal disease, what is maladaptive in one context is actually highly adaptive in another, and the brain is constantly changing—nothing is necessarily permanent.

The harm done by excluding certain disorders from those based in trauma is particularly evident for categories such as schizophrenia and bipolar disorders. In this, an apparent conceptual separation exists that deems experiences like hearing voices or paranoia as "psychotic-like" in those individuals (usually White women) whose trauma is easily recognized as being associated with such experiences, while others (usually Black men) are designated as having a brain disease (i.e., schizophrenia) and truly psychotic for expressing these same internal experiences in a more confusing or symbolic manner (Chap. 3). Perhaps more troubling are those individuals whose trauma is recognized but whose responses to this trauma are dismissed as a personality defect, manipulative, fake, and/ or representative of a multitude of different diseases (i.e., comorbidity; Chaps. 2 and 4).

There is much debate within the mental health field as to how useful, if at all, these diagnoses are and if they actually inform or improve professional interventions. The central purpose of diagnosing and distinguishing alleged disorders is to provide specific treatment recommendations that predictably will help increase positive outcomes and understanding of their etiology (cause); if what is helpful, then, across categories is the same, or if diagnoses actually tell us little beyond the description upon which they are based, are these constructs really doing what they are supposed to do? Is it possible that they are actually preventing us from developing a greater understanding of human behavior?

Often, the classification of a person's suffering has more to do with how well a mental health professional can relate to any particular individual's experiences rather than an objective differentiation of underlying internal processes (e.g., Morrison, 2001). Some practitioners may offer an open and empathic lens to most, yet nonetheless inadvertently ostracize those they do not understand in the process. The concept of dissociative identity disorder (DID), previously known as multiple personality disorder (MPD), is a categorical area in which this segregation and, at times, political discord arise. It is often confused with schizophrenia and/or borderline personality disorder (BPD), due to the fact that they are all describing similar behaviors and experiences, with bitter debates arising both in and out of professional circles on the topic. Are they different? Which ones are real diseases in need of intrusive and coercive biological interventions and which are reactions to trauma? Are some individuals just faking it for attention? What do we really know? And how much do we still not know?

One inadvertent consequence of labeling emotional distress as illness and categorizing different ways of reacting to life as disease is marginalizing people and setting up circumstances that lead to prejudice and discrimination (Chap. 4). People who hear voices or have belief systems that others do not understand are labeled with schizophrenia and said to be suffering a brain disease from which they can never recover and must take debilitating drugs for life in order to function. When such individuals express dissatisfaction with their treatment, they are said to be lacking insight and exhibiting symptoms of their disease. If they express anguish from the traumatic experiences that they believe underlie their distress (which research is now overwhelmingly demonstrating is most often the case, Chap. 6), these traumatic experiences are often dismissed as mere triggers or, worse, delusional. If their voices or fears are recognized as clearly associated with identifiable trauma, such individuals might be diagnosed with BPD or DID, especially if they are female. Yet, when they get angry and/or defensive, they are seen as calculating, difficult, and attention-seeking. If individuals diagnosed with BPD or DID express their anguish through seemingly strange behaviors or enter altered states of consciousness, they are accused of making it up or exhibiting behaviors induced by their therapists (iatrogenesis). These frequent associations are little more than prejudiced stereotypes.

Ongoing efforts to combat stigma by asserting that "mental illness is an illness like any other" are actually associated with *increased* stigma and *increased* efforts to distance oneself from those deemed mentally ill (Read, Haslam, Sayce, & Davies, 2006). On the other hand, providing context to a person's behaviors and emotions not only allows individuals to make meaning of their experience and understand how they make sense given their circumstances, it also locates the problem outside of the person and within relationships. When an emotional problem is conceptualized as internal, as a disease, as a faulty personality, or otherwise, a message is being implied that such a person is innately defective; the problems in the world, in the family, and in society are simply meaningless triggers of an individual deficit rather than the problems themselves. And, if one is a victim of such disease, then it is logical to assume they have no responsibility or control over their behaviors and must, therefore, be controlled by others. By dismissing the life circumstances underlying one's distress and blaming them for having something internally wrong with them, society is, in effect, for many re-creating the traumatic dynamics that led to the distressing experiences in the first place. This is not hyperbole; evidence has demonstrated the traumatizing effects of mental health care for many, with some meeting full criteria for PTSD as a direct result of their treatment experiences (e.g., Mueser, Lu, Rosenberge, & Wolfe, 2010).

Of course, for many others, mental health services may be viewed as life-saving (and for some it also may be both and everything in between!). Certainly, there are numerous individuals helped by traditional mental health interventions and the dedicated individuals who spend their lives assisting others. The subject matter of this book is not about criticizing individual clinicians or negating the beneficent intentions of many mental health professionals. Rather, it is an exploration of the system as a whole, the ideas and assumptions that support the oppressive nature of mental health services, how current treatment practices impact many, especially those who are already marginalized and/or who have experienced severe complex trauma, and what people have found to be helpful, both in and out of the system, when recovering from childhood adversity (Part II). It proposes recommendations and hope for the future by using the voices of those who have had many of the experiences described thus far. It also provides tips on how to find help in the current system, how to develop healthy lifestyles, and other ways in which individuals have learned to find greater life satisfaction (Chap. 10).

WHAT WE SAY MATTERS

The way frameworks are really valuable is when they give people language ... But when frameworks are held as a veil of truth rather than a model, that's where I think a lot of harm happens, and that's where something that starts out as really helpful—I have a language, I can explore this, I can start investing in it, I've got names for it!—People can get stuck in that. And 10 years after they're still using the same model and still using the same framework and they don't know how to shift anything. P5

The way in which language is used to describe something has many implications and can represent forms of power and control (Chap. 3). Some have suggested that the current medicalization of human experience is a form of "colonization" and that reclaiming these experiences is one way to resist an oppressive and discriminatory ideology (e.g., Dillon, 2013). Akin to other civil rights' movements, a mad pride movement exists that, in part, seeks to reclaim terms such as *madness* and to use them in place of the dominant medical terminology.

In an effort to honor these struggles, this book will use the term *madness* wherever possible when referring to emotional distress often described elsewhere as mental illness. It is not equivocal to any particular form of emotional distress and does not insinuate illness, psychosis, insanity, or otherwise. In this same vein, "mental illness" will be in quotes as a qualifier to acknowledge the lack of universal acceptance of this way of viewing emotional distress. Additionally, other medicalized terms or language associated with specific theoretical frameworks or ideology, such as "delusions", "hallucinations", or "alters" will be avoided and, when necessary to use, will be qualified or put in quotes for this same reason.

When discussing belief systems that others might consider to be "delusions", this will be described as having beliefs in conflict with consensus reality (or the reality most people might agree upon). The terms *voices* and *visions* will be used to describe the experience of sensory perceptions without external stimuli (or what some might refer to as "hallucinations"), and *parts* or *self-states* will be used to describe the experience of having depersonalized aspects of the self (or what some may describe as "alters"). Most of these are descriptive terms without assumed meaning behind them. They do not subscribe to any particular school of thought, nor do they insinuate disease, wrongness, or something strange and inexplicable. They are all human phenomena existing on a continuum of severity (Chap. 5).

IMPORTANCE OF UTILIZING "EXPERTS-BY-EXPERIENCE"

And it's about power, and it's about who has it, and so much of the stuff we put down to being 'mentally ill' is actually about completely lacking any social power and not having a voice in any context, and it's about social isolation, and it's about loneliness, and those things don't change until power dynamics change. P5

It has been suggested that an effective integration of the widely varied theories and ideological positions on emotional distress and how to best treat it can be facilitated by including the perspectives and experiential expertise of those who have experienced the phenomena in question (Coons & Bowman, 2001; Milligan, McCarthy-Jones, Winthrop, & Dudley, 2013; Read, 1997). Looking to the subjective experience of service users in developing more effective treatments is a concept that has already proved useful in research on the treatment of "psychosis" (e.g., de Wet, Swartz, & Chiliza, 2015; Walsh, Hochbrueckner, Corcoran, & Spence, 2016), though it remains underutilized in other areas. Moreover, general training courses for psychiatry professionals have been developed by clients in the Netherlands (Boevink, 2012), and non-mainstream recovery-oriented approaches have been developed specifically by experience-based experts (e.g., Randal et al., 2009).

Using experts-by-experience may be most useful when the phenomena appear beyond understanding to professionals and others who have not experienced similar suffering or distress (Bassman, 2001). Furthermore, using experts-by-experience in treatment development and education allows for a less stigmatizing, non-reductionistic understanding and can help lead to more effective means of attitude change (Ng, Pearson, Chen, & Law, 2011). Understanding the personal meaning of how one interprets his or her difficulties allows for a greater focus on respect for the varieties of experience (Geekie & Read, 2009; Randal et al., 2009) without forcing a professional conceptualization. Randal et al. (2009) suggest that professionals come to understand how their customary explanatory models of emotional distress often hinder treatment and contribute to re-traumatization of clients, and how they instead should attempt to enter into the subjective reality of the experiencer.

When suggesting the need for valuing the expert perspective of those with lived experience, it must also be noted that this suggestion is specific to inclusion of such individuals in relatively equal relationships where their view is held in as high regard as those of professionals by "establishing a bond with the [professional] that is based on mutual trust and respect" (P12). This may include having individuals with lived experience helping to develop the questionnaires or design-specific outcomes upon which much of research is based, having them define what is meant by terms such as "recovery", and/or having therapy be client led. Part of the reason for this is that when a person is in an inferior position, as almost every patient is in relation to his or her doctor, that person will often behave or frame things in a way that they believe will please the authority figure. This is especially the case with child abuse victims and others with chronically oppressive experiences, who are basically groomed and programmed to be whomever the authority figure wants them to be. Almost every person who participated in the study upon which this book is based discussed a history of telling their clinicians what they believed the clinician wanted to hear only to realize later just how harmful that very same treatment really was. As stated by one participant:

> I assumed she was right because she was educated. I was not. I was young ... I was still living at home. I was very, very trained to think that anyone that was older than you and educated, you bow. And, it did take me a couple of years after that to really work through some of those things and go 'I actually don't agree.' It really did take me a long time to figure out that I had a right to think differently. P8

Because there have already been critical explorations of mental health care and alternative models of recovery with and about individuals diagnosed with schizophrenia (see, e.g., Mehl-Madrona, Jul, & Mainguy, 2014; Williams, 2012) and, less so, bipolar disorder or BPD (e.g., Cohen, 2005; Mead & Copeland, 2000), I wanted to explore these topics from the perspective of those who identified with the diagnosis of DID. It was curious to me as to whether their stories differ greatly, and, given a trauma-based diagnosis, were they fortunate to receive better and more helpful treatment. I also wanted to explore what they found to be helpful and/or harmful, and if it was any different than those from other diagnostic categories. The entirety of this book is a culmination of the results of my dissertation study combined with first-person perspectives across all diagnostic categories of what is and is not helpful in the healing process. It is an effort to balance the authoritative prescriptions with which we all too often are bombarded from those without the experience under investigation. This includes my own perspective as one who has "been there".

RESEARCH STUDY

As stated previously, there are already numerous first-person accounts and systematic studies providing alternative perspectives on mental health and recovery with individuals who had been diagnosed with schizophrenia, BPD, and/or bipolar disorder, but few exist incorporating the view of individuals diagnosed with DID. Their voices were particularly needed for several reasons: because of the confusion and overlap between these diagnostic categories; the assertions by trauma and dissociative disorder specialists that DID is a distinct trauma-based disorder entirely separate from schizophrenia that requires specialized treatment, even though most of the "symptoms" are indistinguishable; the assertion of most clinicians and psychosis specialists that DID does not exist and is a result of either iatrogenesis (treatment-induced characteristics) or attention-seeking; and the certainty with which most professionals assert the importance of specific types of treatment that are "known" to work.

This book is based on interviews I conducted as part of my doctoral research with individuals from the United States and Australia who identified with a diagnosis of DID (see Table 1.1 for demographic data). All interviews were de-identified and interviewees are anonymous. Individuals who were actively suicidal were not eligible for this study, nor were those who did not speak English, since I speak no other language. For certain, this study was biased towards individuals who were higher functioning and further along in their recovery journey, with most describing themselves as fully recovered. At the same time, most had experienced involuntary hospitalization, four experienced homelessness, and 85% were either under- or unemployed. Additionally, while 77% of the participants had official diagnoses of DID, and all were required to meet a minimum threshold of dissociative experiences as determined by an online questionnaire, this study did not ascertain a diagnosis for purposes of inclusion because of its general lack of validity or reliability.[2]

Although some may suggest that such individuals are not representative of the larger population of individuals diagnosed with DID (and believe me, they have), participants' extensive histories in the mental health system, endorsement of severe and prolonged dissociative and/or "psychotic" phenomena, official diagnoses of DID, and numerous different kinds of treatment experiences are indeed typical of those so diagnosed (see Table 1.2). Sadly, the pessimistic view of many mental health professionals and laypersons alike that individuals who have severe psychotic and/or dissociative experiences cannot ever become fully functioning members of society is too common. I have experienced it first-hand; I have had numerous individuals over the years, including close friends (some of whom happen to also be psychologists) who tell me that I could not possibly have experienced the things I have because, well, I just seem so *normal*. One of the most widely expressed recommendations for professionals

Table 1.1 Demographic data of interview participants ($n = 13$)

	N (%)	Mean (range)
Gender		
Male	0 (0)	
Female	9 (69)	
Genderqueer	2 (15)	
Others	2 (15)	
Race/ethnicity		
Caucasian/White	10 (77)	
Asian/Pacific islander	1 (0.08)	
Hispanic	1 (0.08)	
Others (numerous "due to condition")	1 (0.08)	
Age		36.53 (24–54)
Current employment		
Employed full-time	2 (15)	
Employed part-time	4 (31)	
Unemployed	7 (54)	
Relationship status		
Single	6 (46)	
Separated/divorced	3 (17)	
Partnered	2 (15)	
Married	2 (15)	
Have you previously or do you now experience:		
Hearing voices	10 (77)	
Having visions	8 (62)	
Excessive fear or suspicion of others	8 (62)	
Belief in the paranormal	7 (54)	
Belief in signs of superstitiousness that is outside of your cultural norms	5 (39)	
Excessive social anxiety	10 (77)	

from individuals with lived experience, including all of the participants of this study, is that people can and do recover. And, it is common and probable for them to do so. Would it not seem that those who had gone through such a recovery process would be best suited to advise on what had actually been helpful along the way?

The final research product included a narrative derived from themes, sub-themes, and theoretical concepts based on the interviews conducted. These themes consisted of ideas that were expressed across interviews, and

Table 1.2   Participants' experiences in the mental health system

	N (%)	Mean (range)
Estimated total lifetime years in treatment		8.69 (2.5–22)
Types of therapy experienced[a]		
CBT	8 (62)	
Psychodynamic/"talk therapy"	8 (62)	
Trauma-specific (not DID-specific)	7 (54)	
Multiple psychotropics	6 (46)	
EMDR	5 (39)	
Hospitalizations/AOT	4 (31)	
DID-specific	3 (17)	
DBT	3 (17)	
Sensorimotor/body-focused	3 (17)	
Mindfulness-based	3 (17)	
Hypnosis	3 (17)	
Internal family systems	2 (15)	
Neurofeedback	2 (15)	
Play therapy	2 (15)	
Emotional freedom techniques	2 (15)	
Art therapy	1 (0.08)	
Sexual health counseling	1 (0.08)	
Family therapy	1 (0.08)	
Diagnoses given (known)[b]		5.08 (2 to 8)
DID	10 (77)	
PTSD	9 (69)	
Bipolar	6 (46)	
Psychosis (schizophrenia, schizoaffective disorder, delusional disorder)	6 (46)	
Anxiety (GAD, anxiety NOS)	6 (46)	
Depression	6 (46)	
DDNOS	5 (39)	
BPD	3 (17)	
OCD	2 (15)	
C-PTSD	2 (15)	
Eating disorder	2 (15)	
ADHD	1 (0.08)	
Conversion disorder	1 (0.08)	
Sleep disorder	1 (0.08)	
Initial presenting issue		
Forced treatment for suicidality	3 (17)	
Posttraumatic stress experiences	3 (17)	
Eating disorder	2 (15)	

(continued)

Table 1.2   (continued)

	N (%)	Mean (range)
Psychosomatic issues/medical	1 (0.08)	
Depression	1 (0.08)	
General sense that "something was wrong"	1 (0.08)	
Anxiety	1 (0.08)	
Psychosis	1 (0.08)	

[a]All participants experienced more than one type of therapy; percentages do not add to 100%

[b]Most participants had numerous diagnoses ($\bar{x}$ – 5.08); one participant did not have any official diagnosis due to never using insurance; this was not factored into the overall average

so some unique beliefs or thoughts that were only expressed by a single individual may have been lost in the process. The design was to gain a more generalized narrative as representative of a larger group, rather than a single case study or account. At each stage of the process, a team of researchers had to reach consensus before moving forward to subsequent stages. Additionally, the dissertation supervisor aided in the development of theoretical constructs and the final product had to be presented and defended to a committee of psychologists. This committee included Danielle Knafo, PhD, of Long Island University-Post; Suzanne Philips, PsyD, of Long Island University-Post; and Andrew Moskowitz, PhD, now of Touro College Berlin.[3] This book is based off of the final narrative of the dissertation and will incorporate the voices of the participants throughout, maintaining their voices as central.

Organization of This Book

Trauma and Madness in Mental Health Services is separated into two parts. Throughout each chapter, quotes from the interviews conducted are used to illustrate the principles or suggestions being discussed. In addition, first-person voices from other studies will be incorporated to add strength and support what may be perceived by some as controversial or defiant of accepted facts. Part I is an analysis of the current paradigm of mental health treatment, a brief overview of how the existing understanding of emotional distress came to be, and extensive research findings as they relate to the topic of dissociation, psychosis, and trauma. Much of this background information must be explored and deconstructed if one is to understand the need for a paradigm shift and why so much of what is expressed as helpful has nothing to do with or is in contrast to standard mental health practices. Part II offers helpful suggestions to those who are themselves in the midst of struggling with emotional distress and/or are looking for resources for a loved one.

Chapter 2 explores the history of modern psychiatry as it relates to dissociation and madness beginning in the late nineteenth-century France. The concept of individuals appearing as more than one person, drifting in dream-like awareness, trance states, and other phenomena commonly associated with a diagnosis of DID has been historically documented largely within the context of the schizophrenia diagnosis. Although some researchers and clinicians assert that such phenomena are made up or are the result of certain therapeutic practices, this history tells a different story. Further, it also demonstrates that what is thought of today as "psychotic" is very different than how it once was conceptualized, and how the American culture shaped the current understanding during a time of civil rights protests, feminism, and war.

Chapter 3 discusses the politics involved in mental health and how what is taken for granted as known is not really so. The language that is used is imprecise (as, of course, language generally tends to be) and creates the illusion of difference when there may not be any. For instance, the brain does not know the difference between "trauma" and "severe stress" or "adversity", especially for a young child. Or, how experiences such as hearing voices or having what some determine as bizarre beliefs are deemed "psychotic-like" when conceptualized through a lens of dissociation, but are seen as "psychotic" and the result of brain dysfunction when conceptualized through a lens of schizophrenia, with little beyond opinion and ideology underlying this differentiation. In addition to the ways in which language is used politically, the process of choosing professional members, the ways in which conflicts of interest and careerism create a barrier to openness and curiosity, and how this is all associated with a system based largely on ideological dogma will be discussed.

Chapter 4 explores the *DSM* (American Psychiatric Association, 2013), and the assumptions upon which this manual is based. The diagnostic constructs contained within lack validity and, often, reliability. Further, they are descriptive groupings of behaviors or internal experiences that are decided upon by a group of professionals as existing together. Yet, they are commonly treated as objective entities that exist outside of the opinion of the individual making such a determination. While it is certainly imperative for professionals to have a good understanding of the person they are working with, insistence on correct diagnoses and misdiagnoses makes no sense in this context. Further, many of the lines that are drawn are based on cultural politics, social control, and various biases, such as confirmation bias and expectation bias. Lastly, research on stigma is briefly explored, which demonstrates a clear link between decreased functioning, decreased hope, increased distancing, and decreased empathy with biological and diagnostic frameworks for understanding emotional distress, regardless of intent. Further, these frameworks may actually prevent an individual understanding of the person seeking help and may create more problems than they purportedly solve.

Chapter 5 looks at the continuum of distressing experiences and normalizes what is often judged as inexplicable or bizarre behaviors. What may differentiate those who are clinically diagnosed from those who are not is how much adversity one has experienced and how one expresses his or her internal experiences to others. Many religious factions are based on the idea that suffering is universal and a fact of life, yet we live in a world that tells us we are diseased if we suffer and must seek professional help when in distress. We no longer know how to help each other and be a cohesive social unit. There is often an intuitive understanding of this as it relates to depression or anxiety, but ceases to be considered when looking at phenomena like altered states of consciousness, fragmented or depersonalized parts of the self, fear and paranoia, or other atypical experiences. Having multiple selves has been shown to be universal through theoretical, neurological, and empirical research. Voices and visions, altered states of consciousness, and elaborate unrealistic belief systems are also common, and, in fact, many seek out these experiences to heal from difficult life circumstances. Childhood adversity makes these very human experiences problematic and extreme, but they are not so strange when we see how they exist in everyday life.

Chapter 6 is an overview of the extensive research demonstrating a likely causal relationship between childhood adversity and "severe mental illness". Childhood adversity does not equate with child abuse, though child abuse is one of the most common factors underlying severe emotional distress. Chronic stressors, like relative poverty, extreme dysfunction within the family dynamic, and bullying, have similar effects on the body and mind, as does overt child abuse, though each may be more distinctly related to belief systems and the ways in which one relates with the world. Biological and genetic findings do not conflict with these findings and, in fact, appear to support them. If the problem is childhood adversity, then perhaps that is where intervention, prevention, and research funding efforts need to be directed, regardless of hypothesized diagnoses.

Chapter 7 focuses on the available treatment options and recommendations within the mental health system for individuals with complex trauma, contrasted with what individuals have found to be particularly helpful during their long histories of treatment. Trauma specialists and others have painstakingly elucidated many wonderful tools and therapeutic approaches that are extraordinarily helpful. At the same time, there are areas in which professional recommendations and standard practice conflict with what individuals suggest is actually helpful. Further, what is helpful for one person may be harmful for another, and the need for flexibility and taking an individualized approach to mental health treatment appears to be one of the most important factors in helpful treatment.

Chapter 8 explores how the current coercive, paternalistic, and authoritarian approach to working with individuals in severe distress is harmful and even re-traumatizing for many. A plea for professionals to "stop trying to fix me" and to be able to tolerate the autonomy of the individual was a strong overarching theme arising from every interview conducted, as well as from the larger consumer/ex-patient/mad pride movement. The chapter also explores how some other professionals and professional organizations, such as the British Psychological Society, have developed alternative perspectives in collaboration with individuals with lived experience.

Chapter 9 consists of recommendations for mental health professionals and suggestions on how they and the system as a whole can change in a direction that is more conducive to recovery. This includes utilizing experts-by-experience in research and treatment development, not treating individuals as if they are fragile and in need of rescue, honoring their voices as authorities in their own right, and appreciating the healing power of peer support. Part of the reasoning for this is because it is difficult to understand that which has not been personally experienced, and too often experts-by-training interpret what is important, what overt behaviors mean internally, and what one has or has not experienced in life through the lens of their own lives. This is what has led to accusations of fabrication, attention-seeking, manipulation, delusions (rather than, perhaps, symbolic or metaphorical explanations for real events) and other judgmental dismissals of experience. A therapeutic approach that is most helpful is one that honors the subjective and meets an individual at where he or she is.

Chapter 10 concludes by offering readers suggestions on how to find a helpful therapist, resources on how lifestyle changes can impact one's emotional health, and resources for further information and groups that may be of interest. Although many criticisms of the current mental health system are discussed throughout this book, this does not negate the many helpful clinicians that are working within this system doing the best they can. Therapy can be extremely powerful and life-changing for the better. This chapter is not prescriptive or exhaustive, and readers are encouraged to be attuned to their own good instinct on what they need for their own individual recovery.

Each of these chapters are illustrated and supported by the voices of the interviewees. Of course, this is a small sample of individuals who identify with a particular diagnosis and may not be generalizable to everyone; but, then, that is also one of the major overarching points made throughout the book: Everyone is different, diagnosis or not, and the healing process is one that is highly individual. Healing is about developing healthy relationships, not just with others, but with oneself; the ways in which one does this and with whom cannot be dictated by another, certainly not-me.

NOTES

1. The World Health Organization has done a series of studies beginning in the 1970s evaluating outcomes for "schizophrenia" across countries. They have consistently found that poorer countries (i.e., those countries that have different cultural approaches to emotional distress and rarely react to such conditions with medical interventions) have better outcomes and higher proportions of recovery than richer, more modernized countries (see Jaaskelainen et al., 2013). Yet, in those countries that have since adopted a Western, biomedical approach to emotional distress, the disparity in outcomes has almost disappeared and a poor outcome is now the norm (Karagianis et al., 2009; Whitaker, 2010). See also E. Watters' (2010) *Crazy Like Us*, which documents how the Western view of emotional distress has co-opted other cultures' frameworks for understanding and dealing with such issues, at times, to their detriment.

2. As may already be clear at this point, I do not believe that diagnoses are valid representations of a true construct, nor do I believe that they are ethical to use considering their established lack of validity or reliability (Chap. 4). Therefore, the study conducted did not evaluate for differential diagnosis or comorbidity, but rather for endorsement of specific phenomena including:

feeling like more than one person, extensive memory problems, incidents of possession, and severe depersonalization and derealization.
3. For those interested in the methodological process and the nuances therein can find a copy of the dissertation, entitled "Whose treatment is this anyway? Helpful and harmful aspects of treatment for dissociative identity disorder phenomena?" on *ProQuest* or contact the author directly. What is outlined here is a brief overview geared for the general public who tend to not have a strong understanding of or interest in various quantitative or qualitative methodological procedures. The methods section of the dissertation is almost 30 pages and explains in great detail how participants were selected, how the coding procedure worked, how repeated ideas and themes were developed, the logic behind the use of mixed methods qualitative analysis, and acknowledgment of researcher bias (and the procedures taken to reduce this as best possible).

REFERENCES

American Psychiatric Association. (1980). *Diagnostic and statistical manual of mental disorders* (3rd ed.). Washington, DC: Author.
American Psychiatric Association. (2013). *Diagnostic and statistical manual of mental disorders: DSM-5*. Washington, DC: American Psychiatric Association.
Bassman, R. (2001). Whose reality is it anyway? Consumers/survivors/ex-patients can speak for themselves. *Journal of Humanistic Psychology, 41*(4), 11–35.
Bentall, R. P., Wickham, S., Shevlin, M., & Varese, F. (2012). Do specific early-life adversities lead to specific symptoms of psychosis? A study. *Schizophrenia Bulletin, 38*, 734–740.
Boevink, W. (2012). Towards recovery, empowerment and experiential expertise of users of psychiatric services. In P. Ryan, S. Ramon, & T. Greacen (Eds.), *Empowerment, lifelong learning and recovery in mental health: Towards a new paradigm*. New York, NY: Palgrave Macmillan.
Centers for Disease Control and Prevention (CDC). (2013/2011). *Web-based Injury Statistics Query and Reporting System (WISQARS)*. National Center for Injury Prevention and Control, CDC (producer). Retrieved from http://www.cdc.gov/injury/wisqars/index.html
Cohen, O. (2005). How do we recover? An analysis of psychiatric survivor oral histories. *Journal of Humanistic Psychology, 45*(3), 333–354.
Coons, P. M., & Bowman, E. A. S. (2001). Ten-year follow-up study of patients with dissociative identity disorder. *Journal of Trauma & Dissociation, 2*(1), 73–89.
de Wet, A., Swartz, L., & Chiliza, B. (2015). Hearing their voices: The lived experience of recovery from first-episode psychosis in schizophrenia in South Africa. *International Journal of Social Psychiatry, 61*(1), 27–32.

Dillon, J. (2013, March). Just saying it as it is: Names matter; Language matters; Truth matters. *Clinical Psychology Forum No. 243*: British Psychological Society.

Druss, B. G. (2006). Rising mental health costs: What are we getting for our money? *Health Affairs, 25*(3), 614–622.

Felitti, V. J., Anda, R. F., Nordenberg, D., Williamson, D. F., Spitz, A. M., Edwards, V., … Marks, J. S. (1998). Relationship of childhood abuse and household dysfunction to many of the leading causes of death in adults. *American Journal of Preventative Medicine, 14*(4), 245–258.

Geekie, J., & Read, J. (2009). *Making sense of madness*. New York: Routledge.

Hjorthoj, C. R., Madsen, T., Agerbo, E., & Nordentoft, M. (2014). Risk of suicide according to level of psychiatric treatment: A nationwide nested case-control study. *Social Psychiatry and Psychiatric Epidemiology, 49*, 1357–1365.

Jaaskelainen, E., Juola, P., Hirvonen, N., McGrath, J. J., Saha, S., Isohanni, M., … Miettunen, J. (2013). A systematic review and meta-analysis of recovery in schizophrenia. *Schizophrenia Bulletin, 39*(6), 1296–1306.

Janssen, I., Krabbendam, L., Bak, M., Hanssen, M., Vollebergh, W., De Graff, R., & van Os, J. (2004). Childhood abuse as a risk factor for psychotic experiences. *Acta Psychiatrica Scandinavica, 109*, 38–45.

Karagianis, J., Novick, D., Pecenak, J., Haro, J. M., Dossenbach, M., Treuer, T., … Lowry, A. J. (2009). Worldwide-schizophrenia outpatient health outcomes (W-SOHO): Baseline characteristics of pan-regional observational data from more than 17,000 patients. *International Journal of Clinical Practice, 63*(11), 1578–1588.

Large, M., & Ryan, C. J. (2014). Disturbing findings about the risk of suicide and psychiatric hospitals. *Journal of Social Psychiatry and Psychiatric Epidemiology, 40*(9), 1353–1355.

Mead, S., & Copeland, M. E. (2000). What recovery means to us: Consumers' perspectives. *Community Mental Health Journal, 36*(3), 315–328.

Mehl-Madrona, L., Jul, E., & Mainguy, B. (2014). Results of a transpersonal, narrative, and phenomenological psychotherapy for psychosis. *International Journal of Transpersonal Studies, 33*(1), 57–76.

Milligan, D., McCarthy-Jones, S., Winthrop, A., & Dudley, R. (2013). Time changes everything? A qualitative investigation of the experience of auditory verbal hallucinations over time. *Psychosis, 5*(2), 107–118.

Morrison, A. P. (2001). The interpretation of intrusions in psychosis: An integrative cognitive approach to psychotic symptoms. *Behavioural & Cognitive Psychotherapy, 29*, 257–276.

Mueser, K. T., Lu, W., Rosenberge, S. D., & Wolfe, R. (2010). The trauma of psychosis: Posttraumatic stress disorder and recent onset psychosis. *Schizophrenia Research, 116*, 217–227.

Ng, R. M., Pearson, V., Chen, E. E. Y., & Law, C. W. (2011). What does recovery from schizophrenia mean? Perceptions of medical students and trainee psychiatrists. *International Journal of Social Psychiatry, 57*(3), 248–262.

Parks, S. E., Johnson, L. L., McDaniel, D. D., & Gladden, M. (2010). Surveillance for violent deaths – National Violent Death Reporting System, 16 states. *MMWR 2014, 63*(ss01), 1–33 Retrieved from http://www.cdc.gov/mmwr/preview/mmwrhtml/ss6301a1.htm

Randal, P., Stewart, M. W., Proverbs, D., Lampshire, D., Symes, J., & Hamer, H. (2009). "The re-covery model" – An integrative developmental stress-vulnerability-strengths approach to mental health. *Psychosis, 1*(2), 122–133.

Read, J. (1997). Child abuse and psychosis: A literature review and implications for professionals. *Professional Psychology: Research and Practice, 28*(5), 448–456.

Read, J., Haslam, N., Sayce, L., & Davies, E. (2006). Prejudice and schizophrenia: A revew of the 'mental illness is an illness like any other' approach. *Acta Psychiatrica Scandinavica, 114*(5), 303–318.

Read, J., van Os, J., Morrison, A. P., & Ross, C. A. (2005). Childhood trauma, psychosis, and schizophrenia: A literature review with theoretical and clinical implications. *Acta Psychiatrica Scandinavica, 112*, 330–350.

Walsh, J., Hochbrueckner, R., Corcoran, J., & Spence, R. (2016). The lived experience of schizophrenia: A systematic review and meta-synthesis. *Social Work in Mental Health, 14*(6), 607–624. https://doi.org/10.1080/15332985.2015.1100153

Watters, E. (2010). *Crazy like us.* New York: Free Press.

Whitaker, R. (2010, May). A schizophrenia mystery solved?. *Psychology Today.* Retrieved from https://www.psychologytoday.com/blog/mad-in-america/201005/schizophrenia-mystery-solved

Williams, P. (2012). *Rethinking madness: Towards a paradigm shift in our understanding and treatment of psychosis.* San Rafael, CA: Sky's Edge Publishing.

CHAPTER 2

A History of Dissociation and Madness

It's very important for [mental health professionals] to be educated on the history of their profession ... and the impact Freud has had on this field for the last 100 years. P13

The dissociation and trauma field is one that has brought about a great deal of awareness of the sometimes life-long consequences of developmental trauma and adversity. At the same time, there is much controversy within the larger mental health field as to the legitimacy of some of this research and the treatment practices stemming from the trauma literature. There is no area where this controversy and misunderstanding is more pronounced than that which is associated with dissociative disorder diagnoses, namely, dissociative identity disorder (DID). There is little consensus as to whether DID should even be considered as a valid diagnosis and it is generally not accepted as such within mainstream mental health (Lalonde, Hudson, Gigante, & Pope, 2001). Many researchers and clinicians describe individuals presenting with DID phenomena as attention-seeking and/or enacting behaviors that were essentially created by such individuals' clinicians (Piper & Merskey, 2004).

On the other extreme, there are the steadfast dissociation experts who may ostracize the field by re-labeling and re-classifying phenomena, such as "hallucinations" or "delusions", when trauma is recognized. Additionally, researchers in the dissociative disorders field use terms that are difficult to concretely define (i.e., "alters"; Piper & Merskey, 2005), appear to treat dissociated self-parts as real and separate people (Merckelbach, Devilly, &

© The Author(s) 2018
N. Hunter, *Trauma and Madness in Mental Health Services*,
https://doi.org/10.1007/978-3-319-91752-8_2

Rassin, 2002), and have disagreement among themselves as to what DID even is (Moskowitz, 2011a). The lack of consensus on what constitutes DID, and if it even exists as a true disorder, is actually representative of problems with diagnoses, more generally, and the political and ideological problems rife throughout the mental health field as a whole.

The phenomena and causes of what was formerly known as multiple personality disorder (MPD), now labeled as DID, have been a magnet for controversy throughout history. Their stories are heard in recounting some of the exorcisms in the Catholic Church's history (van der Hart, Lierens, & Goodwin, 1996), the burning of witches in the seventeenth century (Goodwin, 1985; Janet, 1907/1965; Middleton, Dorahy, & Moskowitz, 2008), and many of the early cases of hysteria that launched the modern study of psychology (e.g., Janet, 1901)

According to modern scholars, evidence of altered states of consciousness, amnesia, and severe experiences of feeling not real or detachment from one's body or thoughts (depersonalization) appeared in popular literature and psychiatric research as early as the 1600s (van der Kolk & van der Hart, 1989) and continued to appear in various forms throughout the next several centuries. Franz Anton Mesmer, in the late 1770s, was the first to methodically document cases of individuals with multiple identity states and corresponding amnesia (Middleton et al., 2008). However, DID-like phenomena did not become conceptualized as a specific psychiatric disorder until 1815 (Ellason & Ross, 1995).

Although some suggest that dissociated identity states are the product of over-zealous clinicians and/or an individual effort to get attention, the history of schizophrenia tells us otherwise. From Jean-Martin Charcot's exhibitionist display of women described as hysterical, to the trauma approach of Pierre Janet, women exhibiting seemingly strange and inexplicable behaviors were a central focus of these psychiatrists. The early works of Sigmund Freud were largely in agreement with the trauma approach of Janet. But, as Freud's theories of psychoanalysis expanded and became more popular, the primary role of trauma was submerged by that of purported fantasies and problems attributed to one's personality or character. In tandem, the priorities of medical doctors began to take shape in the asylums and the terms *dementia praecox* and *schizophrenia* became ever more popularized along with a more biological perspective on human nature and distress. The problems with recognizing trauma and humanizing difficult-to-understand behaviors continue to plague the mental health field today, with the DID and schizophrenia factions lying at the center of this conflict and the ongoing nature-versus-nurture debate. So, how exactly did we get here?

WELCOME TO THE CIRCUS

This is not to do with being a freak, thank you very much. P5

In the late nineteenth century, Charcot, one of Freud's early mentors, was the first to systematically study what then was termed hysteria. He would frequently invite other medical professionals to watch the spectacular performances of his hypnotized patients in what has been described as a circus-like atmosphere (Harris, 2005). Women, as it almost never was men, were put on display and seen as objects of fascination, rather than survivors of trauma in need of compassion and understanding. It was not until Janet, Charcot's student, began to recognize the humanness of these women that the role of trauma became the focus of research and examination.

Janet was the first to specifically delineate the link between trauma, dissociation, and various atypical behaviors, as well as to develop a phase-based psychological treatment of remembering and processing unresolved trauma (Howell, 2008; Middleton et al., 2008; van der Hart, Brown, & van der Kolk, 1989). He considered most problems with extreme emotional distress as stemming from early traumatic events that become dissociated, or separated, from conscious awareness (Janet, 1907/1965, 1919/1925). The broad classification of hysteria included numerous and ever-changing experiences, such as: extrasensory perceptions, or "hallucinations" (such as voices), in all senses; amnesia; lack of a stable sense of identity; extreme suggestibility; seemingly odd behaviors or mannerisms; nightmares; unexplainable physical symptoms, such as seizures that lack a physical basis; reenactments of traumatic experiences; flashbacks; paranoia; subjective experiences of possession by outside entities; physical agitation or extreme restlessness; mutism; catatonia; "thought disorder" (or disorganized speech); and/or double personalities (Janet, 1907/1965). Janet stipulated that the limits of classification were vague, but the core of hysteria was the occurrence of existing as if in a dream world, wherein the person loses all contact with reality and has little to no awareness of time, person, or place. This state could last anywhere from a few minutes to up to several years, depending on the complexity. Some current theorists (e.g., Howell, 2008; Moskowitz, Heim, Sailot, & Beavan, 2008; van der Hart & Horst, 1989) suggest that Janet's conceptualization of hysteria likely would have included multiple *DSM* diagnoses, such as borderline personality disorder (BPD), DID, somatization disorders, conversion disorders, major affective disorders, posttraumatic stress disorder (PTSD), histrionic personality disorder, and psychotic disorders.

The treatment of hysteria, according to Janet, included hypnosis for memory retrieval and psychoactive drugs, as well as a phase-based therapy approach that resembles that recommended for complex-PTSD (C-PTSD) today: initial stabilization of crisis, specific work on traumatic memories, and more general work on recovery. While his work with trauma and gradual processing and working through of painful memories may have been groundbreaking, it was Janet's use of hypnosis that created grounds for the rejection of the validity or believability of hysterical phenomena (van der Kolk, Brown, & van der Hart, 1989). Janet, himself, acknowledged that hypnosis could create somewhat artificial behaviors and mental activity, and explicitly expressed concern over the effects this might have on particular individuals (Janet, 1907/1965). He further noted that there was no doubt that observation changes and shapes the expression of underlying experiences but that this did not negate that the phenomena exist. Nonetheless, psychiatry eventually rejected much of Janet's work, presumably based on the potential iatrogenic (clinician-induced behaviors and distress) effects and the improbability of many hysterical presentations (van der Kolk & van der Hart, 1989).

One of the most reputable antagonists of the use of hypnosis was another student of Charcot's, Joseph Babinski (Middleton et al., 2008). He, and other prominent physicians of the time, asserted that hypnosis created symptoms of hysteria and that treatment should only consist of convincing patients of the error in their accusations of abuse and the unreality of their behavioral displays (Middleton et al., 2008; van der Kolk et al., 1989). Janet, on the other hand, expressed that the medical establishment denied the existence of trauma and its effects, focusing too much on the biological to the detriment of the environment (Janet, 1907/1965). This political battle, which greatly influenced the development of Freud's psychoanalytic theories, is not unlike that which is so prevalent today.

FREUD, PSYCHOANALYSIS, AND THE DENIAL OF TRAUMA

Psychoanalysis ... ugh ... Freud ... ugh ... enough said. P13

There is no doubt that Freud and the rise of psychoanalysis transformed both society at large as well as perceptions of individuals suffering emotional distress. He was the first in modern times to convince the world of the powerful healing effects of talking, making popular terms like catharsis, anal retentiveness, repression, defense mechanism, ego, and, of course, penis envy. There was much that was progressive and helpful in what psychoanalysis and some of Freud's theories offered; at the same time, Freud was a controversial figure whose ideas and actions also harmed many, largely through oppression of women and denial of trauma (e.g., Paley, 1979).

Freud studied briefly with Charcot, during which time he also became learned in Janet's theories and techniques. This is reflected in much of Freud's initial work. Like Janet, Freud believed that trauma was the origin of most emotional distress, and that treatment consisted of retrieving and processing these memories (Breuer & Freud, 1895/1960). He recognized that distressing memories may intrude into an individual's conscious awareness through unexplainable physical symptoms, anxiety, or reenactments (wherein one finds his- or herself in the same dynamics or situations repetitively with new people); however, he differed from earlier theorists by introducing the process of repression as a defense against such memories and affects. In his earliest works, Freud's repression was not entirely unlike Janet's dissociation—distressing or overwhelming experiences and emotions become split off or separated from conscious awareness, existing in a separate part of the psyche. As Freud's theories were modified, on the other hand, repression took on new meaning.

The distinction between repression, currently a controversial term, and dissociation is a subject that is imprecise and continues to be debated among scholars.[1] In part, this ongoing debate is due to a lack of consensus on what actually constitutes the construct of dissociation (Dell & O'Neil, 2009; Ford, 2013; Harper, 2011; Nijenhuis & van der Hart, 2011), as well as the interchangeability of the terms *dissociation* and *repression* in many respects (i.e., separation of conscious and unconscious phenomena). What is important here is to know that dissociation, as it was conceptualized by Janet, essentially referred to a trauma-induced splitting of the psyche, while Freud's conceptualization of repression eventually referred to an unconscious process of splitting off intolerable affects, memories, and so on, for the purpose of defense against some internal conflict. Trauma and adversity were no longer central in this process. As Freud shifted away from a framework based on trauma ("seduction theory"), dissociation and its trauma-based associations were replaced by a framework based on unconscious drives (usually sexual in nature), intolerable thoughts or shame, defenses (including repression), and fantasies.

Freud's original "seduction theory" stipulated that all cases of hysteria stemmed from the sexual abuse of a child by an adult figure (Freud, 1896/1954). This was before he changed his contention to the "drive theory", which included the possibility of unconscious fantasies as origins of hysterical symptoms (in other words, the person might just be imagining or fantasizing about being abused; Freud, 1887–1902/1950, 1900/1953). He originally believed that early sexual abuse, usually by the father, was the foundation of somatic, fragmented, and dissociative experiences. Most notably, this was evident in the case study of Anna O., a patient of Freud's colleague Josef Breuer, and perhaps the most famous early case of dissociative phenomena. Breuer and Freud proclaimed that all cases of hysteria were based on some type of hypnotic state of "double-conscience" (Breuer & Freud, 1895/1960), and described Anna O. as being "split into two personalities of which one was mentally normal and the other insane" (p. 46).

On the other hand, accusations of sexual abuse perpetrated by prominent political figures, and seemingly bizarre behaviors allegedly arising from the use of hypnosis were not well-received by the medical establishment (see van der Kolk & van der Hart, 1989). This, along with other possible intellectual and personal motivations, ultimately resulted in Freud's shift away from trauma and dissociation towards unconscious conflicts, fantasies, and repression as the basis of hysteria. It additionally brought about a change from using hypnosis in favor of psychoanalytic techniques, like free association (Freud, 1887–1902/1950).

As psychoanalysis became the dominant paradigm, trauma and dissociation were largely ignored by mainstream psychiatry until the 1980s (Middleton, 2013; Stern, 1996; van der Kolk et al., 1989), even as it was evidenced in war. Soldiers in World War I who had no prior psychiatric difficulties before war were discovered to return with experiences of amnesia (Thom & Fenton, 1920) and severe dissociative phenomena, including personality disintegration and somatic (physical) symptoms (Shephard, 2000). These soldiers not only experienced amnesia for war incidents, but also, at times, complete loss of their past memories (Myers, 1916). In spite of these examples of dissociative and traumatic responses in soldiers, the political and social atmosphere nonetheless supported the denial of childhood trauma and its similar sequelae. As a result, countless individuals who presented with more severe presentations of what was considered hysterical by Janet, were instead blamed, ignored, and/or subjected to the medicalization of their experiences and considered untreatable by psychoanalytic methods[2] (Goldstein, 1978; Middleton et al., 2008; Moskowitz, Heim, et al., 2008; van der Kolk & van der Hart, 1989; Witztum & van der Hart, 2008).

The "Schizophrenias"

At 19, they actually diagnosed me with schizophrenia. And my mother, being scared to death at the time of putting me in a state hospital because of all the stories she heard as a child ... people ending up in mental hospitals, especially state ones ... usually if you went in ... [you] never came out. P10

Numerous developments occurred at the start of the twentieth century in tandem with the rise of psychoanalytic theory. At the time, hysteria and dementia praecox, the precursor to schizophrenia, were two of the major categories of madness. Janet regarded dementia praecox, according to his 1927 paper, *A propos de la schizophrenie* ("Concerning Schizophrenia"), to be characterized by what might be considered the negative symptoms of schizophrenia today: severe social withdrawal into an inner world and engagement in autistic-like behaviors (see Moskowitz, 2008 for a discussion). This was considered by him to be distinctively different from hysterical psychosis, which was dominated by "hallucinations", paranoia, and "delusions." Others have asserted that dementia praecox was a category generally referring to individuals from the lower classes and/or racial minorities (e.g., Metzl, 2010). Freud, however, eventually conceptualized emotional disturbance as existing on a continuum from neurotic to psychotic. In this framework, many of the more severe cases of Janet's concept of hysteria that included prolonged states of unexplainable odd and disorganized behavior were likely considered psychotic in character, rather than hysterical and treatable by psychoanalytic methods.

The category of dementia praecox, then, likely subsumed many, if not most, cases of DID-like presentations that were not dismissed as factitious (Witztum & van der Hart, 2008). Indeed, Car Jung, one of Freud's early students, described dementia praecox as dissociative in nature, with symptoms that included subjective experiences of separate identities and double personalities (Jung, 1909, 1939). Adolph Meyer, one of the most influential people in American psychiatry at the time, believed that a subcategory of dementia praecox cases were unequivocally dissociative and trauma-based (Meyer, Jelliffe, & Hoch, 1911). Specifically, Meyer reported sexual trauma as the source of symptoms such as thought disorder or loose associations that could be reconsidered as the child-like thinking of a traumatized ego state. Emil Kraepelin, the father of the medical model of mental illness, viewed dementia praecox as a biological brain disease (Kraepelin, 1919). Nonetheless, his description of patients was similar to those previously mentioned; he reported on patients who spoke in a child-like manner, experienced other people living inside them, had possession episodes, fugue states, and histories of sexual trauma that were disregarded as delusional. Further, he acknowledged the difficulty in delineating dementia praecox from hysteria in many cases.

This difficulty in diagnostic differentiation and ideological explanatory perspectives continues today. At the time, it also was discovered that many dementia praecox cases were, in fact, cases of encephalitis and other organic diseases treatable by actual medicine. These problems are in general what led Eugen Bleuler to attempt to refine physicians' diagnostic abilities, in the process renaming it *schizophrenia*.

Interestingly, as of the year 2018, it is common to hear or read the rhetoric that schizophrenia is not about split personalities, or that schizophrenia is something entirely different than multiple personalities. Yet, central to Bleuler's theory of schizophrenia were dissociation and processes of splitting within the psyche (Bleuler, 1950). The meaning of the term *schizophrenia* is, in fact, split personality. In some cases, Bleuler's explicit description of splitting included multiple personality states in which the person switched identity, spoke in third person, and had experiences of possession, "hallucinations", and somatic complaints. Schizophrenia was said by him to be an extreme type of splitting, similar to that seen in neuroses, which resulted in amnesia and different personality states governed by explicit emotions and drives. Bleuler stated "These fragments can then exist side by side and alternately dominate the main part of the personality, the conscious part of the patient" (Bleuler, 1950, p. 143).

Apparently, both Freud and Bleuler saw these experiences as existing on a continuum with neuroses, with split personalities sitting towards the extreme end. Bleuler, unlike Freud, considered hypnosis and psychotherapy to be effective treatments for schizophrenia. But, this redefining of dementia praecox to schizophrenia did nothing to end the debating or trouble with differential diagnosis or categorization.

In an effort to further help clinicians easily identify the so-called disease of schizophrenia in their patients, Kurt Schneider (1959) developed a list of symptoms that he believed to be particularly indicative of schizophrenic psychosis, known as Schneiderian first-rank symptoms. In spite of the fact that many have questioned and continue to question their usefulness as a diagnostic tool (American Psychiatric Association, 2011; Peralta & Cuesta, 1999; Silverstein & Harrow, 1978), they still continue to be considered by many as primary indicators of schizophrenia. The specific first-rank symptoms include auditory hallucinations (hearing thoughts aloud, voices commenting, and voices talking about the person in the third person); thought withdrawal, insertion, and interruption; thought broadcasting (having one's thoughts broadcast for others to hear); somatic hallucinations (sensations in or on the body without any physical stimulus); "delusional" perceptions; and made feelings (actions experienced as made or influenced by external agents). Schneider, like Kraepelin, considered schizophrenia to be a biological brain disease, yet he acknowledged that differentiating schizophrenia from soldiers' traumatic reactions to war was difficult (Ross, 2014). In other words, no matter how hard these physicians tried to assert that there was a disease of the mind that was biologically based, none of them could differentiate this so-called disease from individuals' responses to trauma.

After schizophrenia became the conventional terminology, new subcategories based on this term began to arise in the clinical literature to account for the confusing cases of individuals who would present as neurotic, but become psychotic in treatment. Interestingly, it was even alleged that schizophrenia was a result of psychoanalysis itself, or an iatrogenic creation (Federn, 1943), much in the same vein as DID is purported to be currently. Some of these individuals were considered to have *borderline schizophrenia* (Deutsch, 1942; Howell, 2008), while others were described by terms such as *latent psychosis* (Federn, 1943), *pseudoneurotic schizophrenia* (Hoch & Cattell, 1959; Hoch & Polatin, 1949) and a re-emergence of the term *hysterical psychosis* (Hollender & Hirsch, 1964; Spiegel & Fink, 1979). These were cases of individuals who were said to fluctuate from being floridly psychotic to spontaneous recovery (Spiegel & Fink, 1979), or whose psychotic experiences and apparently delusional reactions were allegedly masked by prominent neurotic symptoms, such as anxiety, depression, or phobias (Connor, Nelson, Walterfang, Velakoulis, & Thompson, 2009; Simko, 1968).

Another example of schizophrenia being a term that described individuals experiencing severe dissociation are case studies published during the middle of the twentieth century. Frieda Fromm-Reichmann (1948) stated: "The schizophrenic's problem is not as much that thought or feeling is barred from awareness, but that he is swamped by, from the observer's viewpoint, unconscious material which breaks through the barriers of dissociation" (p. 267). In fact, Fromm-Reichmann's successful psychoanalytic treatment of a so-called "schizophrenic" patient whose presentation of significant dissociative phenomena was indicative of a diagnosis of DID was epitomized in Joanne Greenberg's popular semi-autobiographical novel *I Never Promised You a Rose Garden* (see Sar & Ozturk, 2009; Sperry, 1996; van der Hart et al., 1996).

Repressed ego states in the "schizophrenic" patient were described by Paul Federn as being child-like, independent, and isolated from other states (Federn, 1943). Harold Searles (1965/1986) wrote about overt switching of identity states in his patients, and considered dissociated "doubles" of the self as a specifically schizophrenic defense that allowed the person to remain unaware of unacceptable emotions and experiences. He further described two intertwined types of schizophrenia: the *non-differentiated type*, which was characterized by withdrawal, apathy, flat affect (lack of emotions), and monotonous, stereotyped interpersonal relational styles, and the *non-integrated type*, which was characterized by one person being made up of several different personality fragments that were each dissociated from the other and which allowed the person to be floridly, psychotically paranoid in one moment only to appear calm and lucid in the next.

Further, Harry Stack Sullivan also deemed dissociation to be a central defense in people diagnosed with schizophrenia (Sullivan, 1962). He wrote on the personification of various parts of the personality (Sullivan, 1954), *schizophrenic dissociation* as a defense, and spontaneous recovery from dream-like states (Sullivan, 1962). Gregory Bateson, who developed the double-bind theory of schizophrenia,[3] believed that dissociative phenomena, such as amnesia, hypnotic experiences, and alterations in personality, were fundamental to the idea of schizophrenia (Bateson, Jackson, Haley, & Weakland, 1956). And, lastly, every case described in R. D. Laing's seminal *The Divided Self*, a book attempting to make madness understandable, could be described as a person experiencing a range of dissociated (or divided) self-states. In exemplifying the prototypical "schizophrenic" personality structure, Laing (1960/2010) describes a person for whom memory is "patchy", stating:

> In Julie, each partial system could be aware of objects, but a system might not be aware of the processes going on in another system which was split off from it. For example, if in talking to me, one system was 'speaking', there seemed to be no overall unity within her whereby 'she' as a unified person could be aware of what this system was saying or doing. (p. 190)

Although it is clear that the categories of schizophrenia and DID are based on generally the same dissociative phenomena, they currently exist as distinctly different diagnostic categories. While the term *schizophrenia* refers specifically to a "split psyche" and early presentations were descriptive of dissociative individuals, DID and schizophrenia suddenly became defined as separate, unrelated disorders in 1980. There has yet to be any serious effort within mainstream psychiatry to understand how, or more importantly *if*, these are truly separate syndromes[4]; an illustration of only one of many problems with the *DSM*.

Dissociating Madness

> My personal beliefs are that it's all a crock of shit … it's more common for men to do this, it's more common for trauma victims to do that, or it's more common for someone with schizophrenia to do X—it doesn't add up. It's not an excuse for a behavior, it's not any kind of basis that you should be using as a baseline so that you can work off, I don't think. I find it rather ridiculous. P8

What once was captured by the term *hysteria* during the time of Janet was broken down, with the publication of the *DSM-III* (American Psychiatric Association, 1980), into numerous, seemingly arbitrary categories which were declared to be distinctly different illnesses with different causes, treatments, and prognoses. Essentially, responses to trauma, adversity, and problematic family dynamics became reclassified as diseases of the brain, genetic flaws of the mind or disordered personalities that were isolated from context and ostensibly disconnected by distinct diagnostic boundaries. As will be further discussed in Chaps. 3 and 4, this largely occurred along ideological lines and appears to be impacted greatly by biases based on gender, race, and socioeconomic status. The most common of these broken-down categories are: schizophrenia, DID, BPD, and PTSD.

Schizophrenia, long considered by many to be a dissociative breakdown in the psyche and treatable by psychotherapeutic means, was transformed into a chronic brain disease of savage hopeless individuals requiring biologically intrusive approaches to manage symptoms.[5] At the same time, multiple personality disorder (MPD), which DID was originally called, was included as a new classification considered to be entirely separate from the brain disease of schizophrenia and almost entirely descriptive of middle-upper class White women (as schizophrenia once was; Metzl, 2010). Further, the theoretical character structures considered by psychoanalysts to be the core of all emotional suffering were divided from "real illnesses" into a reprehensible category of personality disorders almost always diagnosed in addition to, rather than instead of, mental illness.

Much of the *DSM* has been influenced by society and popular opinion, rather than on scientific rigor. The inclusion of the diagnosis of MPD was partly due to increased clinical interest that was, to some extent, spurred on by the case of Sybil and the Emmy Award-winning television movie that popularized it (e.g., Nathan, 2011).Though at that time there also was an insurgence of politically-influential traumatized war veterans (van der Kolk et al., 1989) and increasingly numerous publications that reintroduced the study and awareness of dissociation and trauma to mainstream psychiatry (see van der Hart & Dorahy, 2009).

The category of MPD made central the phenomena of shifting identity states, without ever defining what is meant by personality or how a personality controls an individual's behavior. The label itself indicated that an individual had more than one distinct personality, which was said to be confusing and misleading because it was agreed that one does not, in fact, truly have multiple personalities (Ross, 1990). Again, not due to science, but in reaction to criticism and collective opinion, the fourth edition of the *DSM* (*DSM-IV-TR*, American Psychiatric Association, 2000) changed the name to *dissociative identity disorder.*

Despite the name change, the same criticism remained, including the lack of inclusion of more central "symptoms", such as Schneiderian first-rank symptoms, somatic and conversion episodes, depersonalization and derealization, trance states, identity confusion, paranormal experiences, and auditory and visual "hallucinations" (Dell, 2006; Fink & Golinkoff, 1990; Howell, 2011; Kluft, 1987, 2009; Ross, 2011; Ross et al., 1990; Ross & Ness, 2010; Spiegel et al., 2011). Since its inception, the categories of MPD/DID have been criticized by researchers from all areas of interest for being fundamentally flawed and as creating unnecessary confusion, controversy, and misunderstandings (Dell, 2013; Piper, 1994; Sar, Akyuz, & Dogan, 2007). The current edition, *DSM-5* (American Psychiatric Association, 2013) did change the criteria to include a subjective experience of possession and provided a stipulation that others may not observe any switching between personality states. It remains unclear, however, when experiences of possession are "dissociative" versus crossing the line into "psychotic", nor what the difference is supposed to be between switching of states of mind versus "personality". Further, there is no clear explanation as to how one differentiates changing moods and emotional regulation, as is purported to be central to BPD, versus different "personalities" taking control who happen to have different moods and emotions.

Interestingly, an entire section in the *DSM* is dedicated to explaining the differentiation of DID from schizophrenia wherein references are made to voices being "psychotic-like" in DID, even though there is not any evidence ever produced of qualitative differences between voices based on diagnosis (Honig et al., 1998; Moskowitz & Corstens, 2007). This includes the location of the voices as being inside or outside the head (Moskowitz, 2011b). Some have asserted, instead, that this is an effort by the American Psychiatric Association to explain the phenomena of DID while still adhering to a biological framework of conceptualizing schizophrenia, without anything beyond ideology to support this conjecturing (Moskowitz, 2011a; Read, 1997; Ross, 2007).

The result of this dissociation of madness is that comorbidity is the norm, with trauma survivors typically garnering upward of eight to ten diagnoses during their career as a mental health patient. For instance, a study by Ellason, Ross, and Fuchs (1996) found that individuals diagnosed with DID using *DSM-IV* met criteria for an average of 7.3 Axis I disorders ("mental illness"), not including DID, and 3.6 Axis II disorders ("personality disorders"). Some of the most prevalent were 97% major depressive disorder, 79% PTSD, 75% any psychotic disorder, 69% panic disorder, 65% substance abuse, 64% obsessive-compulsive disorder, 56% BPD, 49% avoidant personality disorder, 46% social anxiety disorder, 44% paranoid personality disorder, 42% somatoform disorder, 38% eating disorder, and 27% schizotypal personality disorder. Instead of understanding that people are complex and their reactions to difficult life experiences are also complex, the mental health field, instead, tells such individuals that they have a large number of diseases, each ostensibly requiring a different specific treatment, and, worse, that they have an essentially disordered personality.

As stated by Read, Goodman, Morrison, Ross, and Aderhold (2004), "If we were not constrained by the need for a diagnostic nomenclature we might not need to separate abuse sequelae into seemingly discrete categories, such as PTSD, dissociative disorders, schizophrenia, borderline personality disorder, etc." (p. 24). They suggest that instead these complex and adaptive responses to adversity can be understood as processes that have evolved over time into problematic disturbances in multiple domains. As it stands now, these discrete categories and areas of interest are entrenched in society and in services, with associated stereotypes that serve no one. Sadly, there is much vested interest in maintaining these separations based on specialization, guilds, political power dynamics, and ideological factions that makes it difficult to actually help people cope and heal from human suffering without making them feel defective and othered in the process.

NOTES

1. See (Braude, 2009; Davies, 1996; Freud, 1939/1964; Knafo, 2009; Rivers, 1918; Ross, 2007; Stern, 1996; van der van der Hart & Dorahy, 2009) for different perspectives on this topic. While not discounting the many nuances and philosophical differences, there are two conclusions one may draw: (1) *Dissociation* is a broad term with multiple meanings that includes, but is not limited to, much of what is meant by the term *repression*, and (2) neither term can be separated from the conceptual framework upon which it is based, making comparison of the two a somewhat futile effort.

2. This changing trend was epitomized in Freud's 1905 account of Dora (Freud, 1905/1963). He wrote of a case of a 14-year-old girl who complained of unwanted sexual advances by an adult family friend. Freud described these accusations as projections of Dora's own sexual desires and symptoms of hysteria. When she disagreed, rather than consider the validity of her claims, Freud further blamed her for being disagreeable and vengeful, and declared her untreatable.

3. The double-bind theory of schizophrenia essentially describes a family dynamic wherein an individual is subject to frequent conflicting messages in communication that are mutually exclusive. This creates a lose-lose situation where no matter what the individual does or how he or she responds, it will be wrong. These crazy-making communication styles can be apparent through words, tone of voice, and/or body language. When this dilemma cannot be confronted, the person is said to respond to the confusion by withdrawal and psychic breakdown.

4. There is a group of dedicated scholars (e.g., Connor et al., 2009; Dorahy et al., 2009; Fink & Golinkoff, 1990; Kluft, 1987; Laddis & Dell, 2012; Sar & Ozturk, 2009; Spiegel et al., 2011; Steinberg, Cicchetti, Buchanan, Rakfeldt, & Rounsaville, 1994; van der Hart, Witztum, & Friedman, 1993; Welburn et al., 2003) who have extensively explored *how* these are distinct disorders. But, these authors take for granted that the question of *if* these categories are taxonomically distinct is already answered. This assumption is largely based on the belief that "schizophrenia" is a valid diagnostic category depicting an endogenous brain disease; a long-standing hypothesis that has little evidence to support it, while, on the contrary, the majority of the evidence specifically refutes it (see Zipursky, Reilly, & Murray, 2013 for a review). This leaves the aforementioned authors' conclusions questionable, at best. There are, of course, exceptions to this (e.g., see Morrison, Frame, & Larkin, 2003; Moskowitz, Schafer, & Dorahy, 2008; Ross, 2007 for honest, in-depth debates on this subject), but these alternative efforts to understand this complex issue are certainly not part of mainstream psychiatry.

5. The book *The Protest Psychosis* by Jonathan Metzl outlines a history of schizophrenia from the early 1900s to its modern use. His analysis demonstrates how this diagnosis was once made up mostly of middle- to upperclass White women until the civil rights movement began in the 1960s. In tandem with the rise of power associated with the use of pharmaceuticals, there was a move to quiet the rising voices of Black protestors. At this time, descriptions of individuals diagnosed with schizophrenia were no longer human, but rather depicted animalistic, colored men raging and ranting and in need of immediate tranquilization. To this day, schizophrenia continues to be disproportionately diagnosed in individuals who are of immigrant or minority status.

REFERENCES

American Psychiatric Association. (1980). *Diagnostic and statistical manual of mental disorders* (3rd ed.). Washington, DC: Author.

American Psychiatric Association. (2000). *Diagnostic and statistical manual of mental disorders* (4th ed., text rev. ed.). Washington, DC: Author.

American Psychiatric Association. (2011). Schizophrenia. Retrieved from http://www.dsm5.org

American Psychiatric Association. (2013). *Diagnostic and statistical manual of mental disorders: DSM-5*. Washington, DC: American Psychiatric Association.

Bateson, G., Jackson, D. D., Haley, J., & Weakland, J. (1956). Toward a theory of schizophrenia. *Behavioral Science, 1*(4), 251–264.

Bleuler, E. (1950). *Dementia praecox or the group of schizophrenias* (J. Zinkin, Trans.). New York: International Universities Press, Inc.

Braude, S. E. (2009). The coneptual unity of dissociation: A philosophical argument. In P. F. Dell & J. A. O'Neil (Eds.), *Dissociation and the dissociative disorders: DSM-V and beyond* (pp. 27–36). New York, NY: Routledge.

Breuer, J., & Freud, S. (1895/1960). *Studies on hysteria. Standard edition of the complete psychological works* (J. Strachey, Trans., Vol. 2). London: Hogarth Press.

Connor, K. O., Nelson, B., Walterfang, M., Velakoulis, D., & Thompson, A. (2009). Pseudoneurotic schizophrenia revisited. *Australian and New Zealand Journal of Psychiatry, 43*(9), 873–876.

Davies, J. M. (1996). Dissociation, repression and reality testing in the countertransference: The controversey over memory and false memory in the psychoanalytic treatment of adult survivors of childhood sexual abuse. *Psychoanalytic Dialogues, 6*(2), 189–218.

Dell, P. F. (2006). A new model of dissociative identity disorder. *Psychiatric Clinics of North America, 29*(1), 1–26 vii.

Dell, P. F. (2013). Why the diagnostic criteria for dissociative identity disorder should be changed. *Journal of Trauma & Dissociation, 2*(1), 7–37.

Dell, P. F., & O'Neil, J. A. (2009). Introduction. In P. F. Dell & J. A. O'Neil (Eds.), *Dissociation and the dissociative disorders: DSM-V and beyond* (pp. xxv–xxxiv). New York, NY: Routledge.

Deutsch, H. (1942). Some forms of emotional disturbance and their relationship to schizophrenia. *Psychoanalytic Quarterly, 11*, 301–321.

Dorahy, M. J., Shannon, C., Seagar, L., Corr, M., Stewart, K., Hanna, D., ... Middleton, W. (2009). Auditory hallucinations in dissociative identity disorder and schizophrenia with and without a childhood trauma history: Similarities and differences. *Journal of Nervous and Mental Disease, iii–x*(12), 892–898.

Ellason, J. W., & Ross, C. A. (1995). Positive and negative symptoms in dissociative disorder and schizophrenia. *Journal of Mental and Nervous Disorders, 83*, 236–241.

Ellason, J. W., Ross, C. A., & Fuchs, D. L. (1996). Lifetime axis I and II comorbidity and childhood trauma history in dissociative identity disorder. *Psychiatry, 59*, 255–266.

Federn, P. (1943). Psychoanalysis of psychosis. *Psychiatric Quarterly, 17*, 3–19.

Fink, D., & Golinkoff, M. (1990). MPD, borderline personality disorder and schizophrenia: A comparative study of clinical features. *Dissociation, 3*, 127–134.

Ford, J. D. (2013). How can self-regulation enhance our understanding of trauma and dissociation? *Journal of Trauma & Dissociation, 14*, 237–250.

Freud, S. (1887–1902/1950). *The origins of psychoanalysis*. New York: Basic Books.

Freud, S. (1896/1954). The aetiology of hysteria (J. Strachey, Trans.). In J. Strachey (Ed.), *Complete psychological works* (Vol. 3, Standard ed.). London: Hogarth Press.

Freud, S. (1900/1953). *The interpretation of dreams*. London: Hogarth Press.

Freud, S. (1905/1963). *Dora: An analysis of a case of hysteria*. New York: Collier.

Freud, S. (1939/1964). *Moses and monotheism: Three essays complete psychological works* (Vol. 18, Standard ed.). London: Hogarth Press.

Fromm-Reichmann, F. (1948). Notes on the development of treatment of schizophrenics by psychoanalytic therapy. *Psychiatry: Journal for the Study of Interpersonal Processes, 11*, 263–273.

Goldstein, W. (1978). Toward an integrated theory of schizophrenia. *Schizophrenia Bulletin, 4*(3), 426–435.

Goodwin, J. (1985). Credibility problems in multiple personality disorder patients and abused children. In R. P. Kluft (Ed.), *Childhood antecedents of multiple personality disorders*. Washington, DC: American Psychiatric Press.

Harper, S. (2011). An examination of structural dissociation of the personality and the implications for cognitive behavioural therapy. *The Cognitive Behaviour Therapist, 4*, 53–67.

Harris, J. C. (2005). A clinical lesson at the Salpetriere. *Archives of General Psychiatry, 62*(5), 470–472.

Hoch, P., & Cattell, J. P. (1959). The diagnosis of pseudoneurotic schizophrenia. *Psychiatric Quarterly, 33*, 17–43.

Hoch, P., & Polatin, P. (1949). Pseudoneurotic forms of schizophrenia. *Psychiatric Quarterly, 23*, 248–276.

Hollender, M. H., & Hirsch, S. J. (1964). Hysterical psychosis. *American Journal of Psychiatry, 120*, 1066–1074.

Honig, A., Romme, M., Ensink, B., Escher, S., Pennings, M., & Devries, M. (1998). Auditory hallucinations: A comparison between patients and nonpatients. *Journal of Nervous and Mental Disease, 186*(10), 646–651.

Howell, E. (2008). From hysteria to chronic relational trauma disorder: The history of borderline personality disorder and its links with dissociation and psychosis. In A. Moskowitz, I. Schafer, & M. J. Dorahy (Eds.), *Psychosis, trauma and dissociation: Emerging perspectives on severe psychopathology* (pp. 105–115). West Sussex: Wiley & Sons, Ltd.

Howell, E. (2011). *Understanding and treating dissociative identity disorder: A relational approach*. New York, NY: Taylor and Francis Group, LLC.

Janet, P. (1901). *The mental state of hystericals*. New York: Putnam.

Janet, P. (1907/1965). *The major symptoms of hysteria*. New York: Hafner Publishing Company.

Janet, P. (1919/1925). *Psychological Healing*. New York: Macmillan.

Jung, C. G. (1909). *The psychology of dementia praecox*. New York: Journal of Nervous and Mental Disease Publishing Company.

Jung, C. G. (1939). On the psychogenesis of schizophrenia. *Journal of Mental Science, 85*, 999–1011.

Kluft, R. P. (1987). First rank symptoms as diagnostic indicators of multiple personality disorder. *American Journal of Psychiatry, 144*, 293–298.

Kluft, R. P. (2009). A clinician's understanding of dissociation: Fragments of an acquaintance. In P. F. Dell & J. A. O'Neil (Eds.), *Dissociation and the dissociative disorders: DSM-V and beyond*. New York: Routledge.

Knafo, D. (2009). Freud's memory erased. *Psychoanalytic Psychology, 26*(2), 171–191.

Kraepelin, E. (1919). *Dementia praecox and paraphrenia*. Chicago, IL: Chicago Medical Book Company.

Laddis, A., & Dell, P. F. (2012). Dissociation and psychosis in dissociative identity disorder and schizophrenia. *Journal of Trauma & Dissociation, 13*(4), 397–413.

Laing, R. D. (1960/2010). *The divided self: Existential study in sanity and madness*. London: Penguin Books.

Lalonde, J. K., Hudson, J. L., Gigante, R. A., & Pope, H. G. (2001). Canadian and American psychiatrists' attitudes toward dissociative disorders diagnoses. *Canadian Journal of Psychiatry, 46*, 407–412.

Merckelbach, H., Devilly, G. J., & Rassin, E. (2002). Alters in dissociative identity disorder metaphors or genuine entities? *Clinical Psychology Review, 22*(4), 481–498.

Metzl, J. M. (2010). *The protest psychosis: How schizophrenia became a black disease.* Boston, MA: Beacon Press.

Meyer, A., Jelliffe, S. E., & Hoch, A. (1911). *Dementia praecox: A monograph.* Boston, MA: The Gorham Press.

Middleton, W. (2013). Ongoing incestuous abuse during adulthood. *Journal of Trauma & Dissociation, 14,* 251–272.

Middleton, W., Dorahy, M. J., & Moskowitz, A. (2008). Historical conceptions of dissociation and psychosis: Nineteenth and early twentieth century perspectives on severe psychopathology. In A. Moskowitz, I. Schafer, & M. J. Dorahy (Eds.), *Psychosis, trauma, and dissociation: Emerging perspectives on severe psychopathology.* Wiley-Blackwell: West Sussex.

Morrison, A. P., Frame, L., & Larkin, W. (2003). Relationships between trauma and psychosis: A review and integration. *British Journal of Clinical Psychology, 42,* 331–353.

Moskowitz, A. (2008). Association and dissociation in the historical concept of schizophrenia. In A. Moskowitz, I. Schafer, & M. J. Dorahy (Eds.), *Psychosis, trauma and dissociation: Emerging perspectives on severe psychopathology* (pp. 35–49). West Sussex: John Wiley & Sons, Ltd.

Moskowitz, A. (2011a). Schizophrenia, trauma, dissociation, and scientific revolutions. [Editorial]. *Journal of Trauma & Dissociation, 12*(4), 347–357.

Moskowitz, A. (2011b). Voices, visions and differential diagnosis. *Psychosis, 3*(3), 248–250.

Moskowitz, A., & Corstens, D. (2007). Auditory hallucinations: Psychotic symptom or dissociative experience? *Journal of Psychological Trauma, 6,* 35–63.

Moskowitz, A., Heim, G., Sailot, I., & Beavan, V. (2008). Pierre Janet on hallucinations, paranoia and schizophrenia. In A. Moskowitz, I. Schafer, & M. J. Dorahy (Eds.), *Psychosis, trauma and dissociation: Emerging perspectives on severe psychopathology* (pp. 91–103). West Sussex: John Wiley & Sons, Ltd.

Moskowitz, A., Schafer, I., & Dorahy, M. J. (Eds.). (2008). *Psychosis, trauma and dissociation: Emerging perspectives on severe psychopathology.* West Sussex: John Wiley & Sons, Ltd.

Myers, C. S. (1916). Contributions to the study of shell shock, being an account of certain cases treated by hypnosis. *The Lancet, 190*(65–69), 608–613.

Nathan, D. (2011). *Sybil exposed: The extraordinary story behind the famous multiple personality case.* New York: Free Press.

Nijenhuis, E. R., & van der Hart, O. (2011). Dissociation in trauma: A new definition and comparison with previous formulations. *Journal of Trauma & Dissociation, 12*(4), 416–445.

Paley, M. G. (1979). A feminist's look at Freud's feminine psychology. *The American Journal of Psychoanalysis, 39*(2), 179–182.

Peralta, V., & Cuesta, M. J. (1999). Diagnostic significance of Schneider's first-rank symptoms in schizophrenia. Comparative study between schizophrenic and non-schizophrenic psychotic disorders. *The British Journal of Psychiatry, 174,* 243–248.

Piper, A., Jr. (1994). Treatment for multiple personality disorder: At what cost? *American Journal of Psychotherapy, 48*(3), 392–400.

Piper, A., Jr., & Merskey, H. (2004). The persistence of folly: A critical examination of dissociative identity disorder. Part 1. The excesses of an improbable concept. *The Canadian Journal of Psychiatry, 49*(9), 592–600.

Piper, A., Jr., & Merskey, H. (2005). Reply: The persistence of folly: A critical examination of dissociative identity disorder. *The Canadian Journal of Psychiatry, 50*(12), 814.

Read, J. (1997). Child abuse and psychosis: A literature review and implications for professionals. *Professional Psychology: Research and Practice, 28*(5), 448–456.

Read, J., Goodman, L., Morrison, A. P., Ross, C. A., & Aderhold, V. (2004). Childhood trauma, loss and stress. In J. Read, L. Mosher, & R. P. Bentall (Eds.), *Models of madness: Psychological, social and biological approaches to schizophrenia* (pp. 223–252). Hove: Brunner-Routledge.

Rivers, W. H. R. (1918). The repression of war experience. *The Lancet, 194,* 173–177.

Ross, C. A. (1990). Twelve cognitive errors about multiple personality disorder. *American Journal of Psychotherapy, 44,* 348–356.

Ross, C. A. (2007). *The trauma model: A solution to the problem of comorbidity in psychiatry.* Richardson, TX: Manitou Communications, Inc.

Ross, C. A. (2011). Possession experiences in dissociative identity disorder: A preliminary study. *Journal of Trauma & Dissociation, 12*(4), 393–400.

Ross, C. A. (2014). Dissociation in classical texts on schizophrenia. *Psychosis, 6*(4), 342–354.

Ross, C. A., Miller, S. D., Reagor, P., Bjornson, L., Fraser, G. A., & Anderson, G. (1990). Schneiderian symptoms in multiple personality disorder and schizophrenia. *Comprehensive Psychiatry, 31*(2), 111–118.

Ross, C. A., & Ness, L. (2010). Symptom patterns in dissociative identity disorder patients and the general population. *Journal of Trauma & Dissociation, 11*(4), 458–468.

Sar, V., Akyuz, G., & Dogan, O. (2007). Prevalence of dissociative disorders among women in the general population. *Psychiatry Research, 149*(1–3), 169–176.

Sar, V., & Ozturk, E. (2009). Psychotic presentations of dissociative identity disorder. In P. F. Dell & J. A. O'Neil (Eds.), *Dissociation and the dissociative disorders: DSM-V and beyond* (pp. 535–545). New York, NY: Routledge.

Schneider, K. (1959). *Clinical psychopathology.* New York: Grune & Stratton.

Searles, H. F. (1965/1986). *Collected papers on schizophrenia and related subjects* (Reprint ed.). London: Karnac Books Ltd.

Shephard, B. (2000). *A war of nerves: Soldiers and psychiatrists 1914–1994.* London: Jonathan Cape.

Silverstein, M. L., & Harrow, M. (1978). First-rank symptoms in the postacute schizophrenic: A follow-up study. *The American Journal of Psychiatry, 135*(12), 1481–1486.

Simko, A. (1968). 'Pseudoneurotic schizophrenia' in light of a structural psychopathology. *Der Nervenarzt, 39*(6), 242–250.

Sperry, L. (1996). Dissociative disorders. In L. Sperry & J. Carlson (Eds.), *Psychopathology & Psychotherapy.* New York, NY: Routledge.

Spiegel, D., & Fink, R. (1979). Hysterical psychosis and hypnotizability. *American Journal of Psychiatry, 136*, 777–781.

Spiegel, D., Loewenstein, R. J., Lewis-Fernandez, R., Sar, V., Simeon, D., Vermetten, E., … Dell, P. F. (2011). Dissociative disorders in DSM-5. *Depression and Anxiety, 28*(9), 824–852.

Steinberg, M., Cicchetti, D., Buchanan, J., Rakfeldt, J., & Rounsaville, B. (1994). Distinguishing between multiple personality disorder and schizophrenia using the structured clinical interview for DSM-IV dissociative disorders. *Journal of Nervous and Mental Disease, 182*, 495–502.

Stern, D. B. (1996). Dissociation and constructivism: Commentary on papers by Davies and Harris. *Psychoanalytic Dialogues, 6*(2), 251–266.

Sullivan, H. S. (1954). *The interpersonal theory of psychiatry.* New York: Norton and Company, Inc.

Sullivan, H. S. (1962). *Schizophrenia as a human process.* New York: Norton and Company, Inc.

Thom, D. A., & Fenton, N. (1920). Amnesias in war cases. *American Journal of Insanity, 76*, 437–448.

van der Hart, O., Brown, P., & van der Kolk, B. A. (1989). Pierre Janet's treatment of post-traumatic stress. *Journal of Traumatic Stress, 2*(4), 379–395.

van der Hart, O., & Dorahy, M. J. (2009). History of the concept of dissociation. In P. F. Dell & J. A. O'Neil (Eds.), *Dissociation and the dissociative disorders: DSM-V and beyond.* New York, NY: Routledge.

van der Hart, O., & Horst, R. (1989). The dissociation theory of Pierre Janet. *Journal of Traumatic Stress, 2*, 399–411.

van der Hart, O., Lierens, R., & Goodwin, J. (1996). Jeanne Fery: A sixteenth century case of dissociative identity disorder. *The Journal of Psychohistory, 24*, 1–12.

van der Hart, O., Witztum, E., & Friedman, B. (1993). From hysterical psychosis to reactive dissociative psychosis. *Journal of Traumatic Stress, 6*(1), 43–64.

van der Kolk, B. A., Brown, P., & van der Hart, O. (1989). Pierre Janet on post-traumatic stress. *Journal of Traumatic Stress, 2*(4), 365–378.

van der Kolk, B. A., & van der Hart, O. (1989). Perre Janet and the breakdown of adaptation in psychological trauma. *The American Journal of Psychology, 146*(12), 1530–1540.

Welburn, K. R., Fraser, G. A., Jordan, S. A., Cameron, C., Webb, L. M., & Raine, D. (2003). Discriminating dissociative identity disorder from schizophrenia and feigned dissociation on psychological tests and structured interview. *Journal of Trauma & Dissociation, 4*(2), 109–130.

Witztum, E., & van der Hart, O. (2008). Hysterical psychosis: A historical review and empirical evaluation. In A. Moskowitz, I. Schafer, & M. J. Dorahy (Eds.), *Psychosis, trauma and dissociation: Emerging perspectives on severe psychopathology* (pp. 21–33). West Sussex: Wiley-Blackwell.

Zipursky, R. B., Reilly, T. J., & Murray, R. M. (2013). The myth of schizophrenia as a progressive brain disease. *Schizophrenia Bulletin, 39*(6), 1363–1372.

CHAPTER 3

The Politics of Madness

Health professionals should work more together ... I wish the whole field in general was more accepting towards each other and having a culture where they can actually discuss things ... I'm not sure whether that's just a legacy of the system or whether it's just people with a disposition who enter into the field. I don't know. I find everything a bit kind of archaic and hierarchical and streamlined and I feel like it's counterproductive to the human side of what they're trying to do. P7

Many individuals who are seeking help healing from severe adversity or trauma earlier in life, especially those labeled with diagnoses indicative of "serious mental illness" or a dissociative disorder, have experiences where mental health professionals refuse to work with them, treat them in invalidating and disrespectful ways based on diagnoses, deny their subjective distress and trauma histories, and/or are told their experiences are not real or are efforts to seek attention. Language and the ways in which professionals speak about or describe problems in living create meaning and a specific lens through which a subject is understood. Terms such as *dissociation, delusion, trauma, psychosis,* and others are often thought to have concrete meaning when, in fact, they do not. Granted, language is an imperfect way of expressing complex internal and subjective experiences. Although the language of mental illness provides a framework to describe certain behaviors and emotions, it does so through a particular lens with a specific set of assumptions. Additionally, medicalized and psychologized language tends to give an illusion of exclusive knowledge and separates the lay

© The Author(s) 2018
N. Hunter, *Trauma and Madness in Mental Health Services,*
https://doi.org/10.1007/978-3-319-91752-8_3

person from taking an authoritative stance on his or her own humanity, much in the same way priests did with religious texts in centuries prior (e.g., Whitley, 2008).

Language can be used politically to perpetuate particular belief systems and can create a certain sense of power. The mental health field also maintains authority through selectivity of its members and suppressed dissent. There is a pretense of certainty propagated by leaders in mental health, with oft repeated promises of supporting evidence to be discovered soon; it is taken for granted that their authoritative stance is merited. Despite this political posturing, several areas of concern actually leave much to question, for instance: it is rare for findings to be replicated (Open Science Collaboration, 2015), with only about 3% of journals even being willing to accept articles attempting to repeat previous studies to see if their findings were more than just a fluke (Martin & Clarke, 2017); the peer-review process of journals is biased toward recognizable names and against newcomers or detractors (Bravo, Farjam, Grimaldo Moreno, Birukou, & Squazzoni, 2018), setting up a sort of "good ol' boys' club" dynamic; the rates of authors retracting their studies due to problems or false findings are rapidly rising (Steen, Casadevall, & Fang, 2013); the subjects used in studies are consistently biased (Nielsen, Haun, Kartner, & Legare, 2017) and based on samples that are among the least representative of humans, in general (e.g., Arnett, 2008); spurious and meaningless correlations are frequently reported as exciting new discoveries (see Richardson, 2017); gold-standard "evidence-based treatments" are, on average and *at best*, only helpful for about 25% of people (Shedler, 2015); selective reporting, guild interests, and researcher allegiance heavily bias psychiatric research (Leichsenring et al., 2017; Whitaker & Cosgrove, 2015); and, perhaps most important, with all the purported advances in treatment, the prevalence and long-term outcomes of diagnosable mental disorders has not decreased in the last century (Jorm, Patten, Brugha, & Mojtabai, 2017; Margraf & Schneider, 2016), while disability rates continue to rise exponentially (see Whitaker, 2010 for an analysis on this trend). Yet, the prevailing ideology continues to be praised through distortions and dogmatic replication in widely used textbooks and news sources that rarely question the status quo (e.g., Hunter, 2013).

The biases, career interests, and distortions of information spread to the public and professionals alike stand in the way for vulnerable individuals to find the help they need. There is no room for politics or careerism in helping people who have experienced some of the worst that life has to offer. As proclaimed by one participant: "Talking to somebody about your obstitunami is a privilege … an honor … it's really weird that it's somebody's job, because it's like Holy work … it's really important that [therapists] get that." P4

ON LANGUAGE

I really don't appreciate it, the term *mental illness*. I like to use the term *mentally interesting* … and I don't like *disorder* because … what happened was exquisitely ordered to cause … containment and healing. P4

There's a big difference when you use certain terminology, and *breakdown* will always, always imply that something really not good has happened … and it's not true. It's actually not true. It really needs to be changed … *breakthrough*, because that's what's happening. P10

The emotional impact of the words that are used in communication and, in particular, to describe some phenomena or personal characteristic can be powerful. Entire fields of study are based on the nuances of how language can be used and manipulated to persuade others and/or influence perceptions of power and authority (e.g., Areni & Sparks, 2005; Dillard & Pfau, 2002). Marketers know all too well just how powerful the use of words can be; advertisers know how to use words that affect people outside of conscious awareness (Schrank, 1990). Think of what images and feelings come to mind when hearing words like "groundbreaking", "cutting-edge", "remarkable progress", "precision medicine", or "revolutionary"; these terms regularly fill mental health journals and news stories covering these studies, providing an aura of excitement and pride, with little to no substance behind them.

The language used within the mental health field has a profound impact on the ways in which one understands the meaning of his or her emotional experiences and can even change one's entire sense of identity (e.g., Knight, Wykes, & Hayward, 2003). It additionally has the effect of masking the sometimes assaultive nature of practices, such as saying *electroconvulsive therapy* instead of electrocution of the brain, *Assisted Outpatient Therapy* instead of forced drugging, or implying progress when none is demonstrated by calling something *groundbreaking* despite little evidence of improvement or advancement in treatment or useful knowledge (Newnes, 2016). Words that have the façade of science are used by doctors and other professionals who tend to conceal their essential nature of categorizing societal values through a particular philosophical framework (Jutel, 2009). The term *dissociation*, for example, has no agreed upon definition and means very different things to different people and professionals, based on their particular specialties or vested interests (Dell & O'Neil, 2009; Ford, 2013; Harper, 2011; Nijenhuis & van der Hart, 2011). Yet, it is taken for granted that these medical terms describe some tangible, objective phenomenon that exists in nature, rather than a theoretical construct attempting to explain complex internal experiences and behaviors through a particular theoretical framework.

The diagnosis of BPD, for instance, has been described as little more than an epithet specific to a woman who is perceived as difficult (Vaillant, 1992). In fact, the more educated and trained a professional, the more likely they are to have negative, stereotypical and hopeless views of individuals with this diagnosis (Markham, 2003). A not-uncommon interaction, if perhaps a bit more overt than often allowed, was described by one participant from when she was in "a group setting and ... someone said 'Oh, she's borderline' and the clinicians were like 'No, she can't be. She's not a bitch.'" P13

The phenomenon of hearing things that others do not has numerous different terms associated with it depending on the lens through which one is judging the experiencer. If the person explains the sounds as obviously a replaying of a traumatic experience, then the phenomenon might be called a *flashback*. If this same phenomenon is attributed to radio waves from implanted chips from aliens, it might be called an *auditory hallucination* and a sign of the disease of psychosis. Conversely, if the sounds are attributed to people living inside one's body that are "not-me", they might be described as "psychotic-like" and attributed to an *alter*; however, if the judger is not a believer in DID, then the sounds are instead attributed to the attention-seeking behaviors of BPD and subsequently dismissed. Despite all of these differing perspectives and fancy-sounding names, all are still describing the same experience of simply hearing something that others do not. And, in case there is any question, as already stated, there are no qualitative differences of voices based on diagnoses (Moskowitz & Corstens, 2007), including whether voices exist inside or outside the head (Baumeister, Sedgwick, Howes, & Peters, 2017; Moskowitz, 2011).

Randal et al. (2009) suggest that professionals come to understand how their customary explanatory models of "mental illness" often hinder treatment and contribute to re-traumatization of clients, and how they instead should attempt to enter into the subjective reality of the experiencer.

Using illness language in itself can result in pathologizing and further betraying survivors of trauma (Freyd, 2013).[1] It needs to be recognized that this language is socially and culturally constructed and based on a sociopolitical perception of what is normal (discussion of the validity and use of diagnoses will be further expanded upon in Chap. 4), which in turn gets imposed on a person's subjective sense of distress or ability to cope with adversity in a socially accepted way (e.g., Liegghio, 2016). That is not to say that such frameworks or language are inherently wrong, but rather that they are not inherently right and insisting that they are can be incredibly harmful.

WEEDING OUT THOSE WHO QUESTION

Therapists who are threatened by me has been a huge challenge. I'm smart and I do my own homework and they don't expect that. P5

Doctors are triggering for me, and furthermore, I have found them to generally be rude and arrogant, and as a rule, they do not listen to me; therefore, I do my best to stay away from them. P6

While language tends to create a particular reality and can provide a sense of exclusivity and power, the mental health field also maintains a narrowly focused authority through selectivity of its members and suppressed dissent. Psychiatry and other mental health specializations tend to be focused on conformity and social acceptability (Ventriglio, Gupta, & Bhugra, 2016; Whitley, 2008), serving a central purpose of controlling deviant behaviors and individuals (Hutchinson, 1992), both in service and in education. In many ways, the education process of mental health professionals resembles more a process of indoctrination than that of academic exploration and pursuit.

There are countless stories documenting the suppression and oppression rife within the mental health professions and education process. In 2009, Marcia Angell, former Editor-in-Chief of the *New England Journal of Medicine*, published a controversial book *The Truth About the Drug Companies: How They Deceive us and What to Do About It*, in which she documents the rise of corruption and conflicts of interest within medicine. Despite once being the head of the most prominent and well-respected medical journal in the world, Angell was vilified by her detractors and reframed as a misguided conspiracy theorist when she dared to speak out against the status quo (e.g., Koplewicz, 2011). She, along with other prominent medical professionals, has spoken out about the inflammatory attacks and straw men arguments that appear to result from critical examinations of psychiatric dogma and policy (Steinbrook, Kassirer, & Angell, 2015).

Others have written about losing their funding and jobs for documenting unfavorable findings to the prevailing ideology (e.g., Watson, Arcona, Antonuccio, & Healy, 2014)[2] and being criticized and marginalized within educational programs for dissent (e.g., Hunter, 2015). There have even been instances where researchers were sued by their funding companies for publishing negative results (Bodenheimer & Collins, 2001). It is nearly impossible to get a degree and obtain licensure as a mental health professional without conforming to a strict way of thinking and expressing oneself. Those who question or dare to challenge the status quo are often removed from training, fired from programs, lose or never even receive funding, and/or are not given voice in academic forums (i.e., journals). This suppression of dissent and insistence on conformity is not how science progresses.

SPECIALIZATION, BIAS, AND VESTED INTERESTS

[It] always scares me, when somebody gets too big in the mental health field … When somebody gets too popular in the mental health field, you really have to be careful. P10

Increasing attention has been given to the problems with bias in research and journals' gatekeeping roles on what gets disseminated or not (Hoffman, 2009), the conflicts of interest rife within the mental health field (Paul & Tohen, 2007), the dangers of unwavering adherence to orthodoxy (Murray, 2016), distortions in the peer-review process that appear driven by financial interests (Sudhof, 2016), and how these biases and vested interests may be hindering progress and improvement in outcomes (Gomory, Wong, Cohen, & Lacasse, 2011; Margraf & Schneider, 2016). Physicians frequently overestimate the benefits of their interventions while simultaneously underestimating the risks and harm (Hoffman & Del Mar, 2017; Lilienfeld, Ritschel, Lynn, Cautin, & Latzman, 2014), yet deny that they might be unduly influenced by unconscious motivation and conflicts of interest (Gotzsche, 2015). Funding for research and intervention has shifted away from dealing with social problems and prevention to biological and technical programs (Kolb, Frazier, & Sirovatka, 2000) that have yet to demonstrate any benefit to the understanding or healing of human suffering (Joyner, Paneth, & Ioannidis, 2016). Corporate interests and influence has long been a widely recognized problem throughout all areas of the mental health field (Pachter, Fox, Zimbardo, & Antonuccio, 2007). And, allegiance to a particular specialty (i.e., CBT, psychodynamic) influences outcomes in even the most rigorous of experimental designs, yet, when controlled for, there is little evidence of superiority of particular therapeutic modalities over another (Steinert, Munder, Rabung, Hoyer, & Falk, 2017).

Although one might think that psychology would be the one field where unconscious biases might be acknowledged and considered, it rarely is. Inferential errors are common among clinicians, who tend to attribute client change for the better to intervention effectiveness (illusory causation; Lilienfeld et al., 2014) while change for the worse is attributed to client factors (attributional bias; Batson & Marz, 1979). Diagnoses are conceptual heuristics prone to the same errors inherent in all stereotypes,[3] and their use is directly associated with prejudice and fear (Read, Haslam, Sayce, & Davies, 2006). Increased genetic determinism and "blaming the genes" can be considered as evidence of the *ultimate attribution error* (Pettigrew, 1979), wherein behaviors perceived as problematic by a person from a stereotyped group are considered to be genetically based; at the same time, any positive behaviors are suggested to be exceptions to the rule or due to situational context (i.e., "treatment"). Confirmation biases appear to be rampant, in that researchers and clinicians, unless actively seeking alternative explanations, are likely to observe and take note of behaviors and explanations that fit their preconceived ideas and beliefs (Croskerry, 2002; Garb, 1997; Nickerson, 1998). Another common bias that may arise is an *overpathologizing bias* that describes the tendency for women and minorities to be perceived as requiring more intense and intrusive interventions (Lopez, 2006; Ussher, 2010).

In addition to these common biases to which all humans are prone, power and career goals further contribute to an investment in maintaining the status quo and/or possibly a form of willful blindness. Mental health is an enormous business; in the United States, more money is spent on mental health conditions than any other medical specialty, with an estimated $201 billion spent in 2013 alone and an estimated increase to $280 billion by 2020 (Substance Abuse and Mental Health Services Administration, 2014). More than half of the budget for the American Psychiatric Association is income received directly from pharmaceutical companies, and drug-makers are the most frequent and largest donors of mental health advocacy groups (see, e.g., Harris, 2009). Speaking and consulting gigs for the pharmaceutical industry can earn psychiatrists up to $1 million or more in direct fees per year,[4] and at least 70% of the professionals making up the task force for the *DSM* were tied to pharmaceutical companies (Cosgrove & Krimsky, 2012), raising concerns about corporate interests reflected in practice and policy and accusations of disease mongering (Moynihan, Heath, & Henry, 2002). The incentive for ensuring the medical and biological framework for conceptualizing problems in living is huge.

Willful blindness, or "deliberate harm", is a legal term that describes a process of deliberately avoiding awareness of suggestive evidence and critical facts of possible wrongdoing or harm.[5] When one's job and career identity are dependent on not knowing something, it becomes prudent to remain ignorant. Biological psychiatrists are by no means the only problem in this regard; for instance, specialization in specific disorders or specialty treatments provides marketing tools to sell books, creates a niche for private practice, and allows professionals to book major gigs at increasingly narrowly focused conferences throughout the world, further incentivizing defense of the status quo no matter the problems it may create. If professionals were to acknowledge the complexity of human nature and the direct association of diagnosable mental disorder with adversity and family dynamics, then it would become impossible to deny that there is little specialization beyond helping people with problems in living through human relationship, compassion, attunement, and empathic challenging of behaviors or thoughts. Acknowledging this is an enormous threat to the livelihood of many.

Science Versus Ideology

Behavior and therapies that have been dehumanizing, that have stripped power away from me, that have told me what I must think, must believe, must do ... She was there, as the expert, to re-author my life ... She's an authority figure, she's well-dressed, she's got nice heels, ya know? Half of this is about class. She had money, and prestige, and power, and her opinion counts and I am an absolute bloody nobody who is used to being treated as a nobody by the mental health system and by the welfare system and by everybody else personally that comes into my life. I'm used to being treated as an idiot, I'm used to being treated as just a nobody ... and she said to me "It's not my fault you've failed therapy, and I will be contacting your doctors to let them know you are treatment-resistant and that you are hostile to the process of recovery." P5

An ideology is a set of social or political ideas that serve to explain how society and the world work and how it should change to increase order. Science, on the other hand, is a process of systematically studying the world by utilizing a set of facts or truths that are learned through experiments or observation. The line between the two can become blurred when theories are proclaimed as facts and political ideas distort what is observed. A science becomes an ideology when dissent is suppressed, information is presented in confusing and overcomplicated ways, and when an attitude of omnipotence and authoritarianism is portrayed (Canestrari, 1999). An interesting habit among mental health professionals is to claim pseudoscience for those areas that exist outside the mainstream while continuing to assert their own vested interests as real science (e.g., Herbert et al., 2000; Morgan, 1998). This most frequently can be observed in ongoing debates about CBT versus psychodynamic therapies, neither of which can truly be said to be more effective long-term than the other (e.g., Leichsenring & Steinert, 2017; Steinert et al., 2017), the disparagement of non-professional healing of distress (e.g., Cant & Sharma, 1999) and in comparisons of psychiatry to clinical psychology and/or psychoanalysis.[6]

In general, a true science is open to change and counter-examples, is intent on discovering new ideas even if they contradict currently accepted ones, is open to and encourages criticism and alternative explanations, focuses on replication of results, is humble in its findings and generalizations, and utilizes objective measurement. Conversely, a pseudoscience or faith-based ideology relies on fixed ideas and marginalization of opposition, selectively attends to favorable "discoveries" while ignoring alternative explanations, suppresses criticism and relies on personal attacks and claims of conspiracy, amasses non-verifiable or replicable results, exaggerates claims, and relies on subjective measurements and tautological (circular) reasoning. The mental health field certainly has no shortage of problems concerning conflicts of interest, suppression of dissent, lack of replication, and exaggerated claims.

The ideology of scientism and the biomedical industrial complex (e.g., Gomory et al., 2011) is one based on the faith that understanding the brain will be the key to finally knowing the meaning of life and the nature of consciousness. The central tenet of this ideology is that mental processes, such as emotions, perception, meaning-making, and cognition, are mere facets of neurons and neurochemicals. In this sense, the whole is not greater than its parts. So, for instance, take major depressive disorder (MDD), or depression: it is suggested to be abnormal/not part of the typical human experience, it is bad (evil), it is experienced as a result of faulty neurochemicals, neurons firing inappropriately, and causing the mental experience of sadness and apathy. It has nothing to do with life experience, societal and familial pressures, stress, oppression, patriarchy, or anything else outside of the person; it is simply an errant experience of emotions and behaviors due to short-circuiting in the brain, much like a computer might experience if the wires got crossed. And, if one believes this, despite no testing or evidence to show this postulated brain dysfunction, then faith dictates that an expert is needed to fix this unseen problem. One must seek out a psychiatrist to mediate the mysterious invisible problem and, of course, the only real treatments are those that address this biological problem. Further, if one experiences any kind of mental or physical ailment that does *not* have a scientific-sounding name and an associated pill, the ailment is not taken seriously and often is dismissed. People increasingly can no longer reach out to a friend, change their life, talk to a trusted individual, change their diets, rebel against industrialized and oppressive society, or question those in authority. Just like religion, the people in charge know something no one else can and the evil within us must be quelled. Rather than exorcism, Prozac or Abilify can finally cast out our demons.

In addition to these widely discussed problems, so, too, does the mental health field resort to claims of conspiracy and personal attacks against those in disagreement with the status quo and relies heavily on subjective measurement and tautological reasoning. Again, using the example of depression, this subjectivity and circular reasoning becomes evident. If a person seeks help for feeling sad, lethargic, unmotivated, and experiencing changes in sleep, this person might receive a diagnosis of MDD, a purported brain disease requiring life-long treatment. How does one know that this person "has" MDD? Because they feel sad, lethargic, unmotivated, and has changes in sleep. If the person wants to be really sure, a validated measurement might be given to said person which asks, essentially, if the person is sad, lethargic, unmotivated, and has had changes in sleep patterns. This process is akin to saying "I have a headache", to which a doctor responds "Ah, yes, you have Major Headache Disorder". If asked "How do you know I have Major Headache Disorder?" the answer is "Because you have a headache". And, to make it seem really official, one might be given a questionnaire asking if his or her head hurts. The real stretch is when this gets extrapolated to *explain* things in that "You have a headache *because* you have Major Headache Disorder." This sleight of hand is considered science in the mental health field. What does the person know after visiting the doctor that he or she did not know beforehand? Nothing. Though, for sure, there is the illusion of explanation.

More specifically, this circularity is highly prevalent in the trauma and dissociation field when attempting to support proclamations that "schizophrenia" and "DID" are distinct diseases unrelated and separated along causal lines. This is done by asserting that in DID explanations of phenomena such as hearing voices, feeling possessed, losing touch with reality, and thought/speech disorganization are mediated by dissociation, while in schizophrenia they are not. How do they know? Because they have questionnaires that ask individuals what they attribute these experiences to; if they are explained by *alters*, then they score positive for dissociation, if they are explained by, say, aliens, then they do not. Why is this? Because the people who developed the questionnaire believe that alters are dissociative and aliens are not. Yet, because a questionnaire, biased as it is, says something is so, it suddenly is taken as objective fact and the house of cards continues to rise.

Perhaps the greatest depiction of this circularity and how it allows mental health professionals to maintain omnipotent power is through the use of coercion and symptom mongering. If an individual experiences some kind of crisis or break from reality, any explanation other than that of a medical disease is considered to be wrong and evidence of a lack of insight. If a service user maintains their own explanations of their experience (usually something other than that of illness), they are accused of exhibiting *anosognosia*—meaning, essentially, that the person has a lack of insight into their illness. So, if one disagrees with the clinician that he or she has an illness then that, in and of itself, is proof of their illness.

In response to concerns about the invalid nature of the current diagnostic system, the former head of the National Institute of Mental Health, Thomas Insel, controversially declared a move away from *DSM*-based research (Insel, 2013). While this seems, on its surface, to be an example of following the evidence and adhering to criticism, it actually is anything but. The move is one that is toward a greater focus on brain scan technologies and biological research to develop new categories of illness. Insel, himself, acknowledged that there is no data to actually support this move toward brain-based assessment but, rather, that it is "just beginning" and that it could be considered as "divorced from clinical practice". Although decades of funding dedicated to searching for biomarkers has yielded little, if any, clinically useful results, leaders such as Insel declare that "patients with mental disorders deserve better" and that the answers are just around the corner as technological advances develop. Yet, any noted improvements that have occurred, in general, can be attributed to non-medical prevention efforts (decreased poverty, smoking prevention) and lifestyle changes (e.g., Joyner et al., 2016) begging the question: why are we not moving in this direction?

How can consciousness ever be subject to objective observation and scientific exploration? The idea that the experience of having aliens possessing one's internal faculties versus alternate personalities is somehow representative of different internal processes is mere speculation based on cultural values. How does one claim to know the answer as to how the firing of neurons and transmission of chemicals equals the constructs of love, beauty, or the nostalgia of youth? How does a belief system get reduced to brain processes devoid of context or life experience? Working with individuals who suffer and who have been through adverse experiences is an art, at least according to those very individuals in question, and to reduce it to technology is more illustrative of the values of the current era than it is objective fact. There may be many theories and philosophies, but to claim any as fact is to delude oneself into an illusion of certainty that cannot exist.

Rob Whitley (2008) argues convincingly that psychiatry and clinical psychology have replaced formal religion as a system of beliefs and binding doctrine that dictate the meaning of life with a proselytizing zeal. He demonstrates the parallels between priests and psychiatrists, as well as the missionary work of religion and mental health professionals (euphemistically called "outreach" and efforts to attend to "untreated illness" or "unmet needs"). Of course, as with any religion, people have a right to believe what they find to be resonant with their own experience; the problem begins, however, when people are told that religion is fact and are forced to take on these frameworks and belief systems. It becomes outright tyranny when public policy becomes intertwined with religious belief, and coercive and inhumane practices are justified based on these beliefs.[7]

In his book *Crazy Like Us*, Watters (2010) explores how the missionary-like work of mental health professionals has impacted other societies and colonized their cultural perspectives on human nature. This is of particular concern when considering that non-Westernized cultures have demonstrated better outcomes and increased functioning for diagnoses such as "schizophrenia" (Jablensky & Sartorius, 2008) than do the industrialized countries increasingly imposing their dominant ideologies.

Further, increased adoption of the biomedical ideology is actually associated, overall, with worse outcomes (Firmin, Luther, Lysaker, Minor, & Salyers, 2016), decreased hope, and increased stigma and prejudice (Angermeyer & Matschinger, 2005; Read et al., 2006; Read & Harre, 2001).

The ways in which the prevailing theories and beliefs about the nature of humanity are framed are inextricably enmeshed with cultural values and mythological beliefs of any given age. The "normal" against which all others are currently measured is one that dictates a person show minimal emotion, have little need for social dependency or prolonged attachment to people not presently in one's life, adhere to rigid binary gender roles, obey authority without question or earned trust, avoid questioning accepted ideas or presenting new ideas or methods of action, abide by puritanical ideas of sexuality in a heterosexual context, be strong at all times (unless female, and then not TOO strong), sit still for hours on end with little need for physical activity or movement, support oppressive and violent actions on the part of authority and the State, refrain from engaging in artistic activities that evoke uncomfortable feelings in others, do not rebel, rarely be angry at close others no matter how they behave, and act and communicate in ways that makes sense to mental health professionals. Veer from this and a mental illness (or defective personality) diagnosis is sure to follow. Currently, psychiatry and psychology are the dominant religion, and the *DSM*, aptly described as its bible, with its sisterly doctrine, the International Classification of Diseases (ICD), explain any and all distressing human behaviors in medical and pathological terms so that most, at some point, must come to the reverent mental health professional for saving.

NOTES

1. There also has been discussion of a "biomedical industrial complex" (Relman, 1980) or "psychiatric industrial complex" (Carpenter, 2001) that describes the destructive influence of the medical and corporate interests in defining the nature and causes of psychosocial distress and disapproved behavior. Some have gone so far as equating this with cult indoctrination (Murray, 2009) that is impervious to evidence. See Thomas and Longden (2013) for a theoretical discussion of the resultant harm that comes from technical, medically based frameworks, and their suggestions for non-pathologizing approaches to treating madness in all its varied forms.

2. In 2013, Gretchen LeFever Watson published an article entitled "Shooting the messenger: The case of ADHD" in which she documents a widely publicized incident of losing her job and funding in response to unfavorable results of an evaluation of treatment for "ADHD". She outlines how professionals with strong ties to the pharmaceutical industry engaged in ad hominem attacks while ignoring these results and, instead, increasing potentially harmful drug interventions.
3. See, for instance, Bodenhausen and Wyer (1985) for a discussion on how individuals tend to process complicated information and use judgmental heuristics that underlie problematic stereotypes. Diagnoses, as discussed further in Chap. 4, are conceptual categories that function specifically to allow for quick assumptions and broad classification of complex behaviors and subjective experiences. In general, category-based assessments are closely associated with prejudice and tend to preclude understanding an individual's subjective experience (e.g., Wheeler & Fiske, 2005). See also Jutel (2009) for a discussion of the sociology behind diagnoses and how they function as stereotypes and social tools.
4. It is difficult to ascertain exact numbers for the mental health field, at large, but the project by ProPublica has created an online tool that details drug device or company money paid out between August 2013 and December 2015. The numbers are staggering, with a total of $6.25 billion paid out to 810, 716 doctors and over 1100 teaching hospitals during this time.
5. Willful blindness is a legal concept that allows a defendant to claim a lesser offense than outright negligence or carelessness. This psychological process as it pertains to the court of law was outlined in Margaret Heffernan's book *Willful Blindness: Why We Ignore the Obvious at Our Peril*. Using this term in the context is not necessarily to imply that clinicians or researchers are doing anything illegal, per se, but rather that they are blinding themselves to how their practices and ideological pursuits may be harming people.
6. See Rissmiller and Rissmiller (2006) for a review of various criticisms of biological psychiatry and the current paradigm as it has existed within the so-called antipsychiatry movement. The fact that dissenters or critics are considered to be "anti-" is, in and of itself, an example of how they become marginalized and how language can do this quite simply.
7. It is common in the United States, and other Westernized countries, to allow for forced treatment (i.e., involuntary hospitalization, involuntary ECT, involuntary drugging) if a person is deemed incompetent or a danger to themselves. While some may assert that this is necessary to save lives, this is based on emotion and ideology, not the evidence. For instance, people who are considered to be an imminent threat for completing suicide are often hospitalized against their will, yet, the more involvement with coercive psychiatry, the more likely one is to actually die from suicide (Hjorthoj,

Madsen, Agerbo, & Nordentoft, 2014). Similarly, persons who are considered to be psychotic may also be hospitalized or drugged against their will. Yet, those individuals labeled psychotic who do not comply with standard drugging rituals appear to fare better than those who do (Harrow & Jobe, 2007; Wunderink, Nieboer, Wiersma, Sytema, & Nienhuis, 2013). At the same time, the practice of involuntary interventions is directly associated with PTSD (Mueser, Lu, Rosenberge, & Wolfe, 2010), permanent brain damage (e.g., Breggin, 2003; Moncrieff & Leo, 2010; Morrison, Hutton, Shiers, & Turkington, 2012), prejudice and discrimination (Magliano, Read, Sagliocchi, Patalano, & Oliviero, 2013; Pescosolido et al., 2010; Read et al., 2006), and a profound sense of helplessness (Dillon, 2012). The United Nations has concluded in several reports that involuntary treatment for persons with psychosocial disabilities (i.e., "mental illness") be considered inhumane and that forced drugging, shock, restraint, and seclusion should be banned from all countries, specifically the United States (see Human Rights Council, 2009; Mendez, 2013; Working Group on Arbitrary Detention, 2015).

References

Angermeyer, M., & Matschinger, H. (2005). Causal beliefs and attitudes to people with schizophrenia: Trend analysis based on data from two population surveys in Germany. *British Journal of Psychiatry, 186*(3), 331–334.

Areni, C. S., & Sparks, J. R. (2005). Language power and persuasion. *Psychology and Marketing, 22*(6), 507–525.

Arnett, J. J. (2008). The neglected 95%: Why American psychology needs to become less American. *The American Psychologist, 63*(7), 602–614.

Batson, C. D., & Marz, B. (1979). Dispositional bias in trained therapists' diagnoses: Does it exist? *Journal of Applied Social Psychology, 9*(5), 476–489.

Baumeister, D., Sedgwick, O., Howes, O., & Peters, E. (2017). Auditory verbal hallucinations and continuum models of psychosis: A systematic review of the healthy voice-hearer literature. *Clinical Psychology Review, 51*, 125–141.

Bodenhausen, G. V., & Wyer, R. S., Jr. (1985). Effects of stereotypes on decision making and information-processing strategies. *Journal of Personality and Social Psychology, 48*(2), 267–282.

Bodenheimer, T., & Collins, R. (2001, March 15). The ethical dilemma of drugs, money, medicine. *The Seattle Times.* Retrieved from http://community.seattletimes.nwsource.com/archive/?date=20010315&slug=truth15

Bravo, G., Farjam, M., Grimaldo Moreno, F., Birukou, A., & Squazzoni, F. (2018). Hidden connections: Network effects on editorial decisions in four computer science journals. *Journal of Informetrics, 12*(1), 101–112 https://doi.org/10.1016/j.joi.2017.12.002

Breggin, P. R. (2003). Psychopharmacology and human values. *Journal of Humanistic Psychology, 43*(2), 34–49.

Canestrari, R. (1999). Relationship between ideology and science. *Forum (Genova), 9*(2), 183–190.

Cant, S., & Sharma, U. (1999). *A new medical pluralism? Alternative medicine, doctors, patients, and the state.* London: UCL Press.

Carpenter, M. (2001). It's a small world: Mental health policy under welfare capitalism since 1945. In J. Busfield (Ed.), *Rethinking the sociology of mental health* (pp. 58–75). Oxford: Blackwell.

Cosgrove, L., & Krimsky, S. (2012). A comparison of *DSM*-IV and *DSM*-5 panel members' financial associations with industry: A pernicious problem persists. *PLoS Medicine, 9*(3), e1001190.

Croskerry, P. (2002). Achieving quality in clinical decision making: Cognitive strategies and detection of bias. *Academic Emergency Medicine, 9*, 1184–1204.

Dell, P. F., & O'Neil, J. A. (2009). Introduction. In P. F. Dell & J. A. O'Neil (Eds.), *Dissociation and the dissociative disorders: DSM-V and beyond* (pp. xxv–xxxiv). New York, NY: Routledge.

Dillard, J. P., & Pfau, M. (Eds.). (2002). *The persuasion handbook: Developments in theory and practice.* Thousand Oaks, CA: Sage Publications, Inc.

Dillon, J. (2012). Recovery from 'psychosis'. In J. Geekie, P. Randal, D. Lampshire, & J. Read (Eds.), *Experiencing psychosis.* New York, NY: Routledge.

Firmin, R. L., Luther, L., Lysaker, P. H., Minor, K. S., & Salyers, M. P. (2016). Stigma resistance is positively associated with psychiatric and psychosocial outcomes: A meta-analysis. *Schizophrenia Research, 175*(1–3), 118–128.

Ford, J. D. (2013). How can self-regulation enhance our understanding of trauma and dissociation? *Journal of Trauma & Dissociation, 14*, 237–250.

Freyd, J. J. (2013). Preventing betrayal. [Editorial]. *Journal of Trauma & Dissociation, 14*, 495–500.

Garb, H. N. (1997). Race bias, social class bias, and gender bias in clinical judgment. *Clinical Psychology: Science and Practice, 4*(2), 99–120.

Gomory, T., Wong, S. E., Cohen, D., & Lacasse, J. (2011). Clinical social work and the biomedical industrial complex. *Journal of Sociology and Social Welfare, 38*(4), 135–147.

Gotzsche, P. C. (2015). *Deadly psychiatry and organised denial.* Denmark: People's Press.

Harper, S. (2011). An examination of structural dissociation of the personality and the implications for cognitive behavioural therapy. *The Cognitive Behaviour Therapist, 4*, 53–67.

Harris, G. (2009, October). Drug makers are advocacy group's biggest donors. *The New York Times.* Retrieved from http://www.nytimes.com/2009/10/22/health/22nami.html?_r=2&

Harrow, M., & Jobe, T. H. (2007). Factors involved in outcome and recovery in schizophrenia patients not on antipsychotic medications: A 15-year multifollow-up study. *The Journal of Nervous and Mental Disease, 195*(5), 406–414.

Herbert, J. D., Lilienfeld, S. O., Lohr, J., Montgomery, R. W., O'Donohue, W. T., Rosen, G. M., & Tolin, D. F. (2000). Science and pseudoscience in the development of eye movement desensitization and reprocessing: Implications for clinical psychology. *Clinical Psychology Review, 20*(8), 945–971.

Hjorthoj, C. R., Madsen, T., Agerbo, E., & Nordentoft, M. (2014). Risk of suicide according to level of psychiatric treatment: A nationwide nested case-control study. *Social Psychiatry and Psychiatric Epidemiology, 49*, 1357–1365.

Hoffman, I. Z. (2009). Doublethinking our way to "scientific" legitimacy: The desiccation of human experience. *Journal of the American Psychoanalytic Association, 57*, 1043–1069.

Hoffman, T. C., & Del Mar, C. (2017). Clinicians' expectations of the benefits and harms of treatments, screenings, and tests: A systematic review. *JAMA Internal Medicine, 177*(3), 407–419.

Human Rights Council. (2009, December). Thematic study by the Office of the United Nations High Commissioner for Human Rights on the structure and role of national mechanisms for the implementation and monitoring of the Convention on the Rights of Persons with Disabilities (A-HRC-13-29). *Annual report of the United Nations High Commissioner for Human Rights and reports of the Office of the High Commissioner and the Secretary-General*. Retrieved from http://www.ohchr.org/EN/Issues/Disability/Pages/ThematicStudies.aspx

Hunter, N. (2013). Distortion, bias, and ethical informed consent: Presentations of etiological and treatment factors in abnormal psychology textbooks. *Ethical Human Psychology and Psychiatry, 15*(3), 160–179.

Hunter, N. (2015). Experiences of a 'black sheep' in a clinical psychology doctoral program. In D. Knafo, R. Keisner, & S. Fiammenghi (Eds.), *Becoming a clinical psychologist: Personal stories of doctoral training*. Lanham, MD: Rowman & Littlefield Publishers.

Hutchinson, E. D. (1992). Competing moral values and use of social work authority with involuntary clients. In P. N. Reid & P. R. Popple (Eds.), *The moral purposes of social work: The character and intentions of a profession* (pp. 120–140). Chicago: Nelson-Hall, Inc.

Insel, T. (2013, April). Post by former NIMH director Thomas Insel: Transforming diagnosis. Retrieved from https://www.nimh.nih.gov/about/directors/thomas-insel/blog/2013/transforming-diagnosis.shtml

Jablensky, A., & Sartorius, N. (2008). What did the WHO studies really find? *Schizophrenia Bulletin, 34*(2), 253–255.

Jorm, A. F., Patten, S. B., Brugha, T. S., & Mojtabai, R. (2017). Has increased provision of treatment reduced the prevalence of common mental disorders? Review of the evidence from four countries. *World Psychiatry, 6*, 90–99.

Joyner, M. J., Paneth, N., & Ioannidis, J. P. A. (2016). What happens when underperforming big ideas in research become entrenched? *JAMA, 316*(13), 1355–1356.

Jutel, A. (2009). Sociology of diagnosis: A preliminary review. *Sociology of Health & Illness, 31*(2), 278–299.

Knight, M. T. D., Wykes, T., & Hayward, P. (2003). "People don't understand": An investigation of stigma in schizophrenia using Interpretative Phenomenological Analysis (IPA). *Journal of Mental Health, 12*(3), 209–222.

Kolb, L. C., Frazier, S. H., & Sirovatka, P. (2000). The National Institute of Mental Health: Its influence on psychiatry and the nation's mental health. In R. C. Menninger & J. C. Nemia (Eds.), *American psychiatry after the war* (pp. 207–231). Washington, DC: American Psychiatric Press.

Koplewicz, H. S. (2011, September). Why we need psychoactive meds. *Huffington Post*. Retrieved from https://www.huffingtonpost.com/dr-harold-koplewicz/psychoactive-medication_b_973825.html

Leichsenring, F., Abbass, A., Hilsenroth, M. J., Leweke, F., Luyten, P., Keefe, J. R., ... Steinert, C. (2017). Biases in research: Risk factors for non-replicability in psychotherapy and pharmacotherapy research. *Psychological Medicine, 47*(6), 1000–1011.

Leichsenring, F., & Steinert, C. (2017). Is cognitive behavioral therapy the gold standard for psychotherapy? The need for plurality in treatment and research. *JAMA, 318*(14), 1323–1324.

Liegghio, M. (2016). Too young to be mad: Disabling encounters with 'normal' from the perspectives of psychiatrized youth. *Intersectionalities: A Global Journal of Social Work Analysis, Research, Polity, and Practice, 5*(3), 110–129.

Lilienfeld, S. O., Ritschel, L. A., Lynn, S. J., Cautin, R. L., & Latzman, R. D. (2014). Why ineffective psychotherapies appear to work: A taxonomy of causes of spurious therapeutic effectiveness. *Perspectives on Psychological Science, 9*(4), 355–387.

Lopez, S. R. (2006). Borderline histories: Psychoanalysis inside and out. *Science and Text, 19*, 151–173.

Magliano, L., Read, J., Sagliocchi, A., Patalano, M., & Oliviero, N. (2013). Effect of diagnostic labeling and causal explanations on medical students' views about treatments for psychosis and the need to share information with service users. *Psychiatry Research, 210*(2), 402–407.

Margraf, J., & Schneider, S. (2016). From neuroleptics to neuroscience and from Pavlov to psychotherapy: More than just the "emperor's new treatments" for mental illnesses? *EMBO Molecular Medicine*. https://doi.org/10.15252/emmm.201606650

Markham, D. (2003). Attitudes towards patients with a diagnosis of 'borderline personality disorder': Social rejection and dangerousness. *Journal of Mental Health, 12*(6), 595–612.

Martin, G. N., & Clarke, R. M. (2017). Are psychology journals anti-replication? A snapshot of editorial practices. [Original Research]. *Frontiers in Psychology, 8*(523). https://doi.org/10.3389/fpsyg.2017.00523

Mendez, J. E. (2013, March). Special rapporteur on torture and other cruel, inhuman or degrading treatment or punishment. 22nd session of the Human Rights Council, Agenda Item 3, Geneva.

Moncrieff, J., & Leo, J. (2010). A systematic review of the effects of antipsychotic drugs on brain volume. *Psychological Medicine, 40*(9), 1409–1422.

Morgan, M. (1998, October). Qualitative research: Science or pseudo-science? *The Psychologist, 11*, 481–483.

Morrison, A. P., Hutton, P., Shiers, D., & Turkington, D. (2012). Antipsychotics: Is it time to introduce patient choice? *British Journal of Psychiatry, 201*, 83–84.

Moskowitz, A. (2011). Voices, visions and differential diagnosis. *Psychosis, 3*(3), 248–250.

Moskowitz, A., & Corstens, D. (2007). Auditory hallucinations: Psychotic symptom or dissociative experience? *Journal of Psychological Trauma, 6*, 35–63.

Moynihan, R., Heath, I., & Henry, D. (2002). Selling sickness: The pharmaceutical industry and disease mongering. *BMJ, 324*(7342), 886–891.

Mueser, K. T., Lu, W., Rosenberge, S. D., & Wolfe, R. (2010). The trauma of psychosis: Posttraumatic stress disorder and recent onset psychosis. *Schizophrenia Research, 116*, 217–227.

Murray, R. M. (2016). Mistakes I have made in my research career. *Schizophrenia Bulletin, 43*(2), 253–256.

Murray, T. L. (2009). The loss of client agency into the psychopharmaceutical-industrial complex. *Journal of Mental Health Counseling, 31*, 283–408.

Newnes, C. (2016). *Inscription, diagnosis, deception and the mental health industry.* London: Palgrave Macmillan.

Nickerson, R. S. (1998). Confirmation bias: A ubiquitous phenomenon in many guises. *Review of General Psychology, 2*(2), 175–220.

Nielsen, M., Haun, D., Kartner, J., & Legare, C. H. (2017). The persistent sampling bias in developmental psychology: A call to action. *Journal of Experimental Child Psychology, 162*, 31–38.

Nijenhuis, E. R., & van der Hart, O. (2011). Dissociation in trauma: A new definition and comparison with previous formulations. *Journal of Trauma & Dissociation, 12*(4), 416–445.

Open Science Collaboration. (2015). Estimating the reproducibility of psychological science. *Science, 349*(6251). https://doi.org/10.1126/science.aac4716

Pachter, W. S., Fox, R. E., Zimbardo, P., & Antonuccio, D. O. (2007). Corporate funding and conflicts of interest. *American Psychologist, 62*(9), 1005–1015.

Paul, S. M., & Tohen, M. (2007). Conflicts of interest and the credibility of psychiatric research. *World Psychiatry, 6*(1), 33–34.

Pescosolido, B. A., Martin, J. K., Long, J. S., Medina, T. R., Phelan, J. C., & Link, B. G. (2010). "A disease like any other"? A decade of change in public reactions to schizophrenia, depression, and alcohol dependence. *American Journal of Psychiatry, 167,* 1321–1330.

Pettigrew, T. F. (1979). The ultimate attribution error: Extending Allport's cognitive analysis of prejudice. *Personality & Social Psychology Bulletin, 5,* 461–476.

Randal, P., Stewart, M. W., Proverbs, D., Lampshire, D., Symes, J., & Hamer, H. (2009). "The Re-covery Model" – An integrative developmental stress-vulnerability-strengths approach to mental health. *Psychosis, 1*(2), 122–133.

Read, J., & Harre, N. (2001). The role of biological and genetic causal beliefs in the stigmatization of 'mental patients'. *Journal of Mental Health, 10*(2), 223–235.

Read, J., Haslam, N., Sayce, L., & Davies, E. (2006). Prejudice and schizophrenia: A review of the 'mental illness is an illness like any other' approach. *Acta Psychiatrica Scandinavica, 114*(5), 303–318.

Relman, A. S. (1980). The new medical-industrial complex. *New England Journal of Medicine, 303,* 963–970.

Richardson, K. (2017). GWAS and cognitive abilities: Why correlations are inevitable and meaningless. *EMBO Reports.* https://doi.org/10.15252/embr.201744140

Rissmiller, D. J., & Rissmiller, J. H. (2006). Evolution of the antipsychiatry movement into mental health consumerism. *Psychiatric Services, 57*(6), 863–866.

Schrank, J. (1990). The language of advertising claims. In P. Eschholz, A. Rosa, & V. Clark (Eds.), *Language awareness* (pp. 179–187). New York: St. Martin's Press.

Shedler, J. (2015). Where is the evidence for "evidence-based" therapy? *The Journal of Psychological Therapies in Primary Care, 4,* 47–59.

Steen, R. G., Casadevall, A., & Fang, F. C. (2013). Why has the number of scientific retractions increased? *PLoS ONE, 8*(7). https://doi.org/10.1371/journal.pone.0068397

Steinbrook, R., Kassirer, J. P., & Angell, M. (2015). Justifying conflicts of interest in medical journals: A very bad idea. [Essay]. *British Medical Journal, 350.* https://doi.org/10.1136/bmj.h2942

Steinert, C., Munder, T., Rabung, S., Hoyer, J., & Falk, L. (2017). Psychodynamic therapy: As efficacious as other empirically supported treatments? A meta-analysis testing equivalence of outcomes. *The American Journal of Psychiatry, 174*(10), 943–953.

Substance Abuse and Mental Health Services Administration. (2014). *Projections of national expenditures for treatment of mental and substance use disorders, 2010–2020.* (HHS Publication No. SMA-14-4883). Rockville, MD: Substance Abuse and Mental Health Services Administration.

Sudhof, T. C. (2016). Truth in science publishing: A personal perspective. *PLOS Biology.* https://doi.org/10.1371/journal.pbio1002547

Thomas, P., & Longden, E. (2013). Madness, childhood adversity and narrative psychiatry: Caring and the moral imagination. *Medical Humanities, 39*(2), 119–125.

Ussher, J. M. (2010). Are we medicalizing women's misery? A critical review of women's higher rates of reported depression. *Feminism & Psychology, 20,* 9–35.

Vaillant, G. E. (1992). The beginning of wisdom is never calling a patient a borderline; or, the clinical management of immature defenses in the treatment of individuals with personality disorders. *The Journal of Psychotherapy Practice and Research, 1*(2), 117–134.

Ventriglio, A., Gupta, S., & Bhugra, D. (2016). Why do we need a social psychiatry. [Editorial]. *The British Journal of Psychiatry, 209*(1), 1–2.

Watson, G. L., Arcona, A. P., Antonuccio, D. O., & Healy, D. (2014). Shooting the messenger: The case of ADHD. *Journal of Contemporary Psychotherapy, 44*(1), 43–52.

Watters, E. (2010). *Crazy like us.* New York: Free Press.

Wheeler, M. E., & Fiske, S. T. (2005). Controlling racial prejudice: Social-cognitive goals affect amygdala and stereotype activation. *Psychological Science, 16*(1), 56–63.

Whitaker, R. (2010). *Anatomy of an epidemic: Magic bullets, psychiatric drugs and the astonishing rise of mental illness.* New York: Broadway Paperbacks.

Whitaker, R., & Cosgrove, L. (2015). *Psychiatry under the influence; Institutional corruption, social injury, and prescriptions for reform.* New York: Palgrave Macmillan.

Whitley, R. (2008). Is psychiatry a religion? *Journal of the Royal Society of Medicine, 101,* 579–582.

Working Group on Arbitrary Detention. (2015). Basic principles and guidelines on remedies and procedures on the right of anyone deprived of his or her liberty by arrest or detention to bring proceedings before court. Retrieved from http://www.ohchr.org/EN/Issues/Detention/Pages/DraftBasicPrinciples.aspx

Wunderink, L., Nieboer, R. M., Wiersma, D., Sytema, S., & Nienhuis, F. J. (2013). Recovery in remitted first-episode psychosis at 7 years of follow-up of an early dose reduction/discontinuation or maintenance treatment strategy: Long-term follow-up of a 2-year randomized clinical trial. *JAMA Psychiatry, 70*(9), 913–920. https://doi.org/10.1001/jamapsychiatry.2013.19

CHAPTER 4

The Illness Inquisition

This is not all about … being a freak, thank you very much. P5

In 1487, the *Malleus Maleficarum* was published by members of the Catholic Church in Germany as an authoritative guidebook on how to identify, question, and, ultimately, convict witches. This treatise gave theoretical legitimacy to the act of witch-hunting and endorsed a uniform model of oppression (Stephens, 1998). The scapegoating of people considered odd, non-conforming, or emotionally distressed (mostly women) brought together religious factions as never before, united society on a singular cause, and provided explanations for ailments as widely varying from impotence ("penis theft"; e.g., Smith, 2002) to intense emotional suffering and physical pain.

This guidebook was a major resource during the Inquisition and witch-hunting craze. While modern thinking may lead one to laugh or scoff at its supposed silliness, this book was wildly popular and served as the professional manual for witch hunters for almost three centuries. The endeavor of identifying, classifying, and interrogating witches was highly sophisticated and was the purview of highly educated, elite professionals who would marginalize and officially condemn detractors of their craft. The *Malleus Maleficarum* was used by judges and prosecutors and was printed and reprinted over 13 times throughout the more than 200 years it held persuasion. Once a person was defined as a witch, they often would admit to impossible feats, such as flying on poles, and would behave in bizarre

© The Author(s) 2018
N. Hunter, *Trauma and Madness in Mental Health Services*,
https://doi.org/10.1007/978-3-319-91752-8_4

and frightening ways in accordance with perceived expectations. Similarly, the *DSM* serves as an authoritative manual written by sophisticated, elite, usually White men, providing a guide for identifying and classifying individuals who disturb, who defy social norms, and who are considered to be somehow different.

The detection of witches also included accepted testing methods that were perceived as scientific and used within the legal system to convict and condemn those who failed.[1] Some of these tests included such barbaric practices as being thrown into water to see if they would sink or float ("swimming test"), being subjected to public stripping to examine for blemishes or a "Devil's Mark" that was evidence of partnership with Satan, or pricking the suspect's skin to see if it would bleed or if she would experience pain. Other, less overtly cruel tests, included having suspects recite passages from the Bible; if the person could not do so without error, this was evidence of witchery (as opposed to, say, illiteracy or nervousness). In this same vein, modern tests of "mental illness" include examining if individuals can recite random information that would only be familiar to Western, educated individuals and to communicate in complete and proper sentences as expected by professionals and society; if they fail, as the witches of the past, this can become proof of their defectiveness of mind.[2]

Consistent across time, with both the witches of centuries past and those individuals diagnosed with serious mental illness in the present, the persons most likely to be identified and classified include those in poverty, women and minorities, and individuals with long histories of trauma and oppression (Barstow, 1988; Cassiman, 2008; McDonald, 1997; Middleton, Dorahy, & Moskowitz, 2008). Many individuals were forthcoming in internalizing and accepting their identification as witch, as this was the only framework through which to contextualize their aberrant behaviors and experiences, much in the same way many do so today with their illness labels. As stated by Jackson (1995), "Witch-hunting was a method of behavioural control in which women as victims (in many senses of the word) were themselves participating because they had no other framework of reference" (p. 63).

The mental health paradigm and its professionals have long been described as providing a means through which to maintain control and govern the marginalized (e.g., Penfold & Walker, 1984; Stark & Flitcraft, 1988). In fact, since at least 1980, there has been strong opposition to the *DSM* on the grounds that it largely serves to scapegoat victims of trauma, oppression, and discrimination (Brown, 1992; Unger & Crawford, 1992). One must ask how much has really changed in the last 300 years.

THE *DSM* IS NOT RELIABLE OR VALID

Psych labels, across the board, were harmful. P1

The original *DSM* editions were broadly based on a psychoanalytic model representing proposed *reactions*, realizing the contextual nature of these categories, and were largely used for work within the US Veterans Administration (e.g., Pilgrim, 2014). Due to many factors, including a crisis of legitimacy within the field of psychiatry, leaders pushed to restructure the manual. The goal was to focus less on clinical intuition and more on a hypothesized research-based method of operational definitions of behavior and emotions and increased reliability among professionals (see Wilson, 1993 for a review of this history). There were 106 categories in the first *DSM*, while that number has ballooned to well over 300 in the latest version (*DSM-5*; American Psychiatric Association, 2013). While it may seem to some that the addition of new categories or changes within these manuals was due to scientific discovery, in fact it has much more to do with the competitive and financial demands of professionals, corporations, and health insurance companies (Kinderman, Allsopp, & Cooke, 2017; Mayes & Horwitz, 2005).[3]

The diagnoses currently used by mental health professionals around the world are socially constructed entities, based on a medical model of emotional distress, developed by the American Psychiatric Association in order to conceptualize various hypothetical disease processes that can purportedly lead to specific treatments, predict outcomes and course of illness, and from which generalizations can be made (Frances, 2016; Hare-Mustin & Marecek, 1997; Jablensky & Sartorius, 2008).

People tend to find diagnoses useful because they appear to provide an explanatory model for their distress and offer a language to express subjective experiences. Additionally, there is the belief that they will lead to specific treatments that, in turn, will lead to a predictable outcome. In other words, diagnoses give people a sense of understanding and hope for a concrete fix.

Yet, diagnostic categories lack predictive value (Jablensky & Sartorius, 2008), nor do they tend to provide any tangible clinical usefulness (Hornstein, 2013; Wakefield, 2016). They are generally based on subjective guesswork (Johnstone, 2014) and sociopolitical values and preferences (Wakefield, 2016) and do not appear to be warranted by scientific research (Caplan, 1995). Simply put, diagnoses do not do what they are designed to do (Bentall, 2003; British Psychological Society, 2013; Deacon, 2013).

There is evidence that the reliability ratings for some categories have been increased since adopting this system in 1980. This means that, given a particular set of "symptoms" and a specific presentation, professionals tend to agree on what label seems fitting for the given individual. Of course, just because professionals agree does not necessarily mean that the thing they agree upon is an objective fact or a true entity that exists in nature, especially when considering the indoctrination process one had to have gone through to be in a position to make such a decision in the first place (see Chap. 3). Even with these "improvements", however, reliability ratings continue to be little better than random chance. Put another way, even though leaders of psychiatry (Kraemer, Kupfer, Clarke, Narrow, & Regier, 2012) give the impression that there is "cause for celebration" (p. 14), clinicians rarely agree upon a diagnosis for any given individual, and those that they do agree upon are usually descriptive of only one or two phenomena (i.e., panic disorder is a category simply describing a person who has panic attacks).

For example, although schizophrenia is definitively described as a debilitating brain disease in need of drugs for life, and is associated with loss of liberty and autonomy for most, even under the most stringent and controlled setting where doctors explicitly know they are being tested on their ability to agree with one another, the reliability ratings are demonstrated to be between 0.39 and 0.50 (Regier et al., 2013). In every other field of medicine, this rating is considered poor and unacceptable (e.g., Cicchetti, 1994). Yet, as is typical of leaders in the mental health field, a simple change of words (from "poor" to "good", in this instance) gives an illusion of acceptability and progress. The result is people being told, with certainty, that they have a disease sometimes considered worse than cancer without any proof and with agreement among clinicians as to the diagnosis only slightly better than flipping a coin.

More important than reliability is validity; a diagnosis is considered scientifically valid if it is consistent across time, allows for prediction of course and treatment, is distinct from other diagnoses, and describes what it is designed to describe (i.e., a true disease that exists in nature). Further, in order for a diagnosis to be valid, it first must be reliable, which most are not. Diagnostic categories based on the *DSM* also lack validity in all of these areas. They do not map onto any specific underlying biological abnormality (e.g., Owen, 2014), nor do they lead to an increased understanding of why a person is suffering or how they can be helped (e.g., Jablensky & Sartorius, 2008). In terms of reliability and validity, the *DSM* is no better than it was in the 1970s and is not supported by the broader research (Vanheule, 2017).

To illustrate the *DSM*'s lack of validity as it pertains to madness more generally, take the categories of schizophrenia, DID, PTSD and BPD. These are purported to be separate diseases of vastly different etiology (causes), prognoses, and treatments. Schizophrenia is said to be a mostly genetic brain disease requiring biological interventions, with little hope for recovery (see, e.g., Zipursky, Reilly, & Murray, 2013 for a critical review). DID is a disorder closely related to PTSD, acknowledging a traumatic etiology, and thought to be treatable by psychological means, often only by those who specifically specialize in this area (e.g., Brand et al., 2012). Somewhere in between, BPD exists as a disorder of the character of a person based partly on genetics and partly on trauma, requiring both biological and psychotherapeutic interventions (e.g., Crowell, Beauchaine, & Linehan, 2009), and is mildly associated with recovery (almost all who are diagnosed are thought to no longer meet the criteria eventually, though apparently it takes about 30 years for that to happen; Paris, Brown, & Nowlis, 2001). And all of these suppositions exist despite the fact that there still is not a single objective identifiable marker for any *DSM*-defined category, as acknowledged by the head of the most recent *DSM* (Kupfer, 2013).

These categories are highly overlapping and little, if any, notable differences between these diagnoses exist, depending on who is doing the judging. What differences do emerge largely appear to reflect levels of severity and biases based in culture, gender, and race. For instance, some say that DID is a severe form of BPD, with little differentiating the two (e.g., Lauer, Black, & Keen, 1993) and both existing as a disorder of disorganized attachment and dissociation (e.g., Howell, 2008). BPD is also considered to possibly be a severe mood disorder (see Parker, 2014 for a discussion) or, more specifically, part of a bipolar spectrum (Smith, Muir, & Blackwood, 2004). BPD also regularly co-occurs with a diagnosis of either bipolar or schizophrenia spectrum disorders (Gunderson et al., 2006; Kingdon et al., 2010). Similarly, up to 75% of individuals with a DID diagnosis also meet the criteria for a psychotic disorder (Ellason, Ross, & Fuchs, 1996), while approximately 60% of individuals diagnosed with schizophrenia meet the criteria for a dissociative disorder (Ross & Keyes, 2004).

Almost half of all individuals diagnosed with PTSD score as high as those diagnosed with DID on a scale measuring severe dissociation (Carlson, Dalenberg, & McDade-Montez, 2012; Carlson & Putnam, 1993), and approximately 80% of those who meet the criteria for DID also meet the criteria for PTSD (Ellason et al., 1996). Because so many individuals meet the criteria for PTSD, there have been several articles suggesting that a dissociative subtype of PTSD may subsume many cases of DID (Lanius et al., 2010; Lanius, Brand, Vermetten, Frewen, & Spiegel, 2012; Wolf et al., 2012), while there is actually very poor statistical support for PTSD and dissociative disorders as separate disorders (Dalenberg & Carlson, 2012).

Schizophrenia also has been described as possibly being a severe form of PTSD (e.g., Coughlan & Cannon, 2017; Morrison, 2001), with "hallucinations" and "delusions" representing severe forms of flashbacks and reenactments, and negative symptoms as avoidance and numbness. At the same time, others purport that DID is a mild form of schizophrenia or that there should be a dissociative subcategory of schizophrenia that would likely consume many cases of DID (Vogel, Braungardt, Grabe, Schneider, & Klauer, 2013). This suggested category may represent up to half of all individuals diagnosed with schizophrenia (Ross & Keyes, 2004). It is common for individuals diagnosed as psychotic to report amnesia for identity and other personal facts when presenting for emergency services, yet this is considered to be a primary feature of DID (Foote & Park, 2008; Parks, Hillard, & Gillig, 1989). At the same time, individuals diagnosed with DID frequently present initially with psychotic experiences, such as disorganized thinking, "hallucinations", and lack of reality testing. Researchers from both the psychotic and dissociative disorder fields have suggested the need for combining the study of both (Read, 1997; Varese, Udachina, Myin-Germeys, Oorschot, & Bentall, 2011) and conceptualizing DID as lying on a continuum with schizophrenia (Morrison, Frame, & Larkin, 2003; Ross & Keyes, 2004; Sar et al., 2010). Schizophrenia has also been theorized to be a severe form of depression (Upthegrove, Marwaha, & Birchwood, 2017), while others have pointed out the extraordinary overlap between schizophrenia and anxiety disorders (e.g., Pokos & Castle, 2006). Of note, anxiety disorders and depressive disorders also tend to co-occur at such high rates so as to suggest that they may not exist as separate disorders either (e.g., Jacobson & Newman, 2017).

With so much overlap among these ostensibly distinct diseases, what actually makes them different? Psychotic disorder diagnoses are most common among poor and minority individuals (Feisthamel & Schwartz, 2009; Neighbors, Trierweiler, Ford, & Muroff, 2003; Nguyen, Huang, Arganza, & Liao, 2007) and among minority immigrants (but not White immigrants; Kirkbride et al., 2017). Conversely, bipolar disorder and most personality disorder diagnoses are more commonly given to White individuals compared to Black persons (Barnes, 2008, 2013; Coleman et al., 2016; McGilloway, Hall, Lee, & Bhui, 2010). In fact, the mental health system has been described as a form of institutional racism due to both diagnostic and treatment practices (e.g., Wade, 1993).

Bipolar disorder, DID, and BPD are also typically diagnoses given primarily to women (Altshuler et al., 2010; Hartung & Widiger, 1998; Sansone & Sansone, 2011; Shaw & Proctor, 2005; Wasserman, McReynolds, Ko, Katz, & Carpenter, 2005; Widiger & Spitzer, 1991). This may be partly due to the fact that women tend to experience more "positive symptoms", such as paranoia, extrasensory perceptions, disorganization, and affect dysregulation (Abel, Drake, & Goldstein, 2010; Cotton et al., 2009; Zhang et al., 2012), which are thought to be indicative of these diagnoses (Moskowitz, Read, Farrelly, Rudegeair, & Williams, 2009; Read, van Os, Morrison, & Ross, 2005). At the same time, men are more likely to experience apathy, blunted emotions, and withdrawal (Goldstein, 1995; Willhite et al., 2008), considered to be more indicative of psychosis or schizophrenia (Moskowitz, 2008). It appears as though race, gender, and socioeconomic status can indicate a particular diagnosis better than any underlying pathology, while pathology, itself, is often considered as anything straying from the ideal of the White, upper-class, Western man (Barnes, 2013; Bussey & Bandura, 1999; Cook, Warnke, & Dupuy, 1993; Hurst & Genest, 1995; Neighbors, Jackson, Campbell, & Williams, 1989; Salokangas, Vaahtera, Pacriev, Sohlman, & Lehtinen, 2002).

Liotti and Gumley (2008) consider DID, schizophrenia, PTSD, and BPD to all be variations along a continuum of having a fragmented sense of self (much like R.D. Laing purported 60 years ago and Janet did over a century ago). Others have returned to Freud's original suggestion that emotional distress lies on a continuum from neurotic to psychotic without distinct diagnostic boundaries (e.g., Kelleher & Cannon, 2016). The linking factors of neurodevelopmental changes from trauma (Read et al., 2005), disorganized attachment, and dissociation (Howell, 2008), and the vastly overlapping phenomenology support the idea that these are not, in fact, distinctly separate disorders and can all possibly be treated with trauma-informed therapeutic practices with specific techniques geared toward specific complaints (e.g., Bentall, 2003).

For an individual facing the prospect of any of these various diagnoses, DID and PTSD are the only ones to acknowledge trauma and the adaptive nature of distressing experiences. Conversely, being given a diagnosis of schizophrenia appears to be sufficient to increase the likelihood one will die from suicide (Fleischhacker et al., 2014). To be sure, diagnoses give the illusion, for many, of explanation, understanding, and redemption from judgments of moral defectiveness. If one is sick, then he or she is not bad. But, why must a person be considered as defective at all? Are the only choices really to be bad or sick? What if we used more accurate descriptive terms that do not blame victims? Like "sexual abuse survivor syndrome" or "gaslighting parent reaction". Imagine how different society and professionals would look at and interact with such individuals.

Please Do Not Make Assumptions

It is important to listen and not automatically assume that you know what's going on with the other person. [Don't] be so quick to jump to judgments or assumptions, and listen. I think that it's really important. I think that if he [first therapist] would have done that, ya know, maybe he could've helped me ... just don't assume that you know who a person is, what they're dealing with, what they've been through, ya know, people aren't like one dimensional. P6

Ok, there's something else that doesn't help. Don't assume! P9

One of the most helpful things, according to people who have been there, is for clinicians to be open to the subjective, without making assumptions. Yet, the very purpose and result of diagnoses is precisely that: to make assumptions. Diagnoses are heuristics, categories with stereotyped associations, and depending on one's theoretical orientation will subsequently lead to a particular set of assumptions based on these stereotypes. This would be helpful if these categories were valid, but they are not. Rather, they act as any other stereotype does and frequently result in erroneous extrapolations and judgmental reactions on the part of mental health professionals, intentional or not. It is common for individuals with more serious diagnoses to experience chronic invalidation, dismissiveness, and harmful treatment within the mental health system. Of course, some individuals' behaviors can certainly elicit responses from others that are not always helpful, but this does not negate the discriminatory and prejudicial role that diagnoses often play.

Once assumptions are made, confirmation and expectations biases will often give the illusion that the assumption was correct when, in fact, the assumption is often shaping behaviors and beliefs. As stated by one participant: "You're almost evoking 'borderline' behavior by coming and leading a group or leading a therapy session with the assumption that this is who the client, this is who I am ... Yeah, I'm gonna act a little bitchy if you treat me like that without getting to know me" (P13). People want to please their therapists, especially individuals who have experienced significant trauma, and will frequently lie (Blanchard & Farber, 2016) and behave in a manner they believe is expected by authority.

DID is a controversial diagnosis and often purported to be iatrogenic, or developed as a result of the treatment process itself (see, e.g., Gillig, 2009), and so such individuals are frequently accused of lying, faking, and/or as needing to be ignored until they present as doctors want them to. The assumption that individuals who are "schizophrenic" present with consistent, overt phenomena and a complete inability to have insight leads to dismissiveness toward those who minimize, hide, or vary in their outward presentation. At the same time, individuals diagnosed with BPD are said to be "attention-seeking" or "manipulative" when disclosing voice-hearing or other purportedly psychotic phenomena. An article by Desai, Summers, and Bunker (2013) demonstrated the serious adverse outcomes that can arise from confusion over and discriminatory biases associated with diagnoses. Specifically, these authors discussed the problem of practitioners in the UK dismissing persons who were considered to have BPD as not really being psychotic, or having "pseudohallucinations", and as being "manipulative", "attention-seeking", and/or eschewing responsibility by faking these phenomena. These individuals are then denied services as a result. Forcing a diagnostic box around a person is often impossible without also forcing untrue characteristics and making false assumptions that are based on prejudiced heuristics and self-fulfilling prophecies.

In addition, as already discussed, the constructs in the *DSM* value stereotypically Western, male traits while pathologizing traits more typically associated with other genders or cultures (Addis & Mahalik, 2003; Bussey & Bandura, 1999; Cook et al., 1993). The ethnocentric assumptions rife within the current mental health paradigm result in the denial of the legitimacy of variations in the expression of distress, despite nods to the importance of "cultural sensitivity". For instance, other cultures may express distress through physical ailments (China), burning soles of the feet (Sri Lanka), or semen loss (India; Marecek, 2006; Watters, 2010). Disturbingly, race and ethnicity are the most significant predictors of a diagnosis of schizophrenia (Barnes, 2013; Fabrega, 1996; Feisthamel & Schwartz, 2009; Foulks, 2004). This is not just a matter of "misdiagnosis";

inherent in diagnostic procedures are assumptions that deny cultural differences of expressing distress (e.g., Neighbors et al., 1989). Diagnoses are nothing if not a set of assumptions based on judgmental stereotypes and heuristics based on the values of one specific culture.

Difference in Severity Does Not Equate with Difference in Kind

Then there's gonna be a different way that person's gonna get treated. Period. That person will always be seen as a schizophrenic. Always be seen as a bipolar. Always be seen as just DID. Always be seen as just all the 20 million *DSM* [disorders], which is really another joke, ya know? That's the sad part. P10

In the late nineteenth century, Janet theorized a continuum of traumatic responses that included ever-changing variations in expression of distress. Freud later postulated a continuum from neurotic to psychotic, with the borderline in between classifying most individuals who were not considered to be pervasively psychotic (Kernberg, 1975). But, with the development of the *DSM*, what once was considered a continuum of responses to trauma and adversity was suddenly broken down into arbitrary categories theorized to represent hypothetical diseases.

It has been argued by many that there is no sharp distinction between emotional distress considered "normal" or "neurotic" and those considered "psychotic" (Freeman & Garety, 2003), and that psychosis, PTSD, BPD, DID, and other problems in living may be considered as similar and integral phenomena that exist as part of a spectrum of responses to trauma (McWilliams, 2015; Morrison et al., 2003). What appears to often differentiate a diagnosis of schizophrenia versus PTSD, for instance, is cultural acceptability of meaning-making processes and severity of experience rather than any objective difference in the underlying process (Morrison, 2001). It is a common experience for trauma survivors to be reinforced in their fragmented view of themselves by being led to believe that somehow only some of their emotional experiences are related to trauma, while others are "disease". This is often expressed through messages that one has "co-morbid disorders" or that some problems are due, for instance, to a disordered personality, while others are due to the biological genetic disease of, say, bipolar disorder. The political and ideological literature throughout the trauma and dissociative disorder fields is consistent with this fragmented way of conceptualizing problems; this is not only a problem of biologically oriented psychiatrists.

It may be suggested by some that diagnoses are important because they aid in the process of determining appropriate drug treatment. Aside from the already discussed lack of predictive validity for *DSM*-defined categories, generally, psychotropic drugs actually do not have any such specificity to diagnoses (Moncrieff, 2008, 2013). For example, it has consistently been demonstrated that antidepressants essentially act as numbing agents and are rarely more effective than active placebo (e.g., Kirsch et al., 2008). Cocaine and other stimulants can enhance learning and help with focus and attention, whether one meets the criteria for ADHD or not (Lakhan & Kirchgessner, 2012; Moncrieff, 2013). Similarly, neuroleptics—euphemistically called "antipsychotics"—are tranquilizers that result in sedation and indifference, and are more useful for behavioral control rather than any specific effect to psychosis (De Fruyt & Demyttenaere, 2004; Dubin & Feld, 1989; Moncrieff, 2013).[4] Similar to pain relievers, just because a drug "works" does not mean that there is some underlying, specific disease process that it is working upon.

Likewise, trauma-informed, normalizing treatment interventions, including exposure therapy (Frueh et al., 2009), mindfulness-based (Chien & Thompson, 2014), narrative (Mehl-Madrona, Jul, & Mainguy, 2014), and other non-medication-based (Morrison, Hutton, Shiers, & Turkington, 2012) approaches, have been found to be helpful across diagnostic categories, including schizophrenia, suggesting diagnoses are inadequate in determining what will or will not be helpful in treatment above the considerations of the specific problems any individual may be uniquely presenting with. Further, according to psychiatrist Mark Zimmerman (2015, July 24), practices with a specific focus on delineating "accurate" diagnoses may not be important in determining helpful treatment. Rather, what is more important is to take an individualized, collaborative, trauma-informed approach that is attuned to individual needs without making assumptions and considering the person's subjective experiences as real and something to be respected.

MANUFACTURING DISEASE

And just seeing yourself as not sick, ya know, I think that's so important, to, ya know, not attach a stigma to whatever diagnoses you or the other parts of yourself might get, and to be able to say: "Yeah, yeah, I deal with that, but I'm doing ok, and everybody has stuff that they have to deal with and it's normal to some degree." P3

I can't wait till these words are out of our culture, out of our world all together. P10

Although claiming to be neutral as to what supposedly causes madness, the *DSM* and its diagnoses are based upon a biomedical model (Erlandsson & Punzi, 2016). Essentially, by medicalizing human suffering, the problems in society, within families, and the general injustice of the world go ignored. Instead, the problems are placed inside individual brains. If context is considered, it becomes a mere trigger of an underlying disease rather than the problem in itself.

By calling an experience of human suffering a "disorder" or "mental illness", a particular frame of understanding as to the cause and nature of the distress is implied. In his book *Manufacturing Depression: The Secret History of a Modern Disease*, Greenberg (2010) describes how human suffering and melancholy have been packaged by scientists, and, in turn, through brilliant marketing suggests that one needs an expert intervention (often a biological one), that one's suffering has nothing to do with the external world, and that it is up to the individual to fix themselves. Pharmaceutical marketing and psychiatric guilds have been ingenious in their ability to turn almost every physical and emotional experience of being human into a disease, coming up with a convoluted name, and then concluding that the only remedy is expert intervention and drugs. This creation of diseases not only serves pharmaceutical interests; rather, guild and professional interests of psychiatrists, psychologists, social workers, counselors, and all the hundreds of boutique organizations made for every specialty imaginable all exist, thrive, and receive profit from this disease paradigm.[5] Certainly, most professionals are well-intentioned and enter into the field to be helpful; this does not negate, however, the inherent biases that arise from professional and career interests and the resultant unconscious motivation to protect the status quo for the purpose of self-preservation.

Regardless of how any individual clinician may conceptualize a person's distress, the current paradigm under which all mental health professionals operate is one that is conceived through a medical ideology with a medical classification system (Caplan, 1995; Frances, 2016). Terms such as "symptoms" are used to describe human behaviors and emotions (Hare-Mustin & Marecek, 1997), while many categories are associated with words like "neurological", "genetic predisposition", and "illness", despite no known biological abnormality to be specifically associated with any *DSM*-defined category (e.g., Kupfer, 2013).

An example of how contrived this disease-mongering process can truly be is exemplified in the history of the so-called antidepressant Prozac. In 1987, Prozac was first marketed as a breakthrough drug that could target chemical imbalances in the central nervous system and brain that caused the disease of major depressive disorder. This was the first selective serotonin reuptake inhibitor (SSRI), and the marketing proved wildly successful: in its first year, sales in the United States were around $350 million with an eventual peak at $2.6 billion a year (see McLean, 2001). Due to commercials and the "education" of prescribers directly by pharmaceutical representatives, the idea that people who were sad and depressed had chemical imbalances in their brains became common parlance. So how is this an example of manufacturing a disease? There is no such thing as a chemical imbalance that is known to cause some identifiable disease called depression. In fact, leaders within psychiatry have called the chemical imbalance theory an "urban legend" that was never taken seriously by "well-informed psychiatrists" (Pies, 2011). An entire society was led to believe in a disease known to be caused by neurochemical imbalances as a direct result of a genius marketing scheme, and nothing more (see also Schultz & Hunter, 2016 for a review).

SOCIAL CONTROL

> And it's about power, and it's about who has it, and so much of the stuff we put down to being mentally ill is actually about completely lacking any social power and not having a voice in any context, and it's about social isolation, and it's about loneliness, and those things don't change until power dynamics change. P5

In addition to providing profits for individual and corporate interests, as well as providing a certain ideology regarding the meaning of life and suffering, diagnoses and the illness paradigm provide a convenient means by which to control society. Religion has traditionally been the vehicle through which those in power could justify the status quo and convince people to believe in the fairness and legitimacy of social institutions and structures (Jost et al., 2013). In many ways, the mental health field operates in the same way as religion has in times past (e.g., O'Neill, 1986).

During the time of slavery, those who dared to seek freedom and run for their lives were diagnosed with the mental illness *drapetomania*, the cure for which was a master kind enough to provide "work" (e.g., Bynum, 2000). No one could understand why a slave would not wish to kneel before his master, so it made perfect sense that a disease must be causing him to run away. In later years, Black individuals were once again pathologized for daring to fight back against a racist society when schizophrenia became rebranded from a disorder mostly descriptive of middle-class White women to that of the angry, violent Black man (Metzl, 2010). One need only look at any advertisement during the 1960s for neuroleptic drugs, which almost exclusively featured an animalistic looking Black man clearly needing to be tranquilized like a feral dog.

In current society, children who are incapable of sitting for hours at a time, focusing quietly on boring materials with little-to-no exercise or opportunities to just be children, get diagnosed as having the neuro logical disease of ADHD, even though many neurologists keep telling the public that no such disease exists (e.g., Saul, 2014). Psychologist Bonnie Burstow (2017) has called the drugging of children, particularly for the purpose of behavioral control, a direct act of child abuse. Women have been subjected to interventions geared toward making them more docile and sexually submissive since at least the fifth century BC (Tasca, Rapetti, Carta, & Fadda, 2012) and frequently are pathologized for their reactions to sexual abuse and rape that might disturb others.[6] And, anti-authoritarians or people who rebel against the status quo are often diagnosed with oppositional defiant disorder and prescribed tranquilizing and numbing drugs to force conformity and compliance.[7] People who defy binary conceptualizations of gender and are sad about their discomfort with not fitting in are diagnosed with the mental illness gender dysphoria, said to be distinct from the disease process of depression. And, if one is prone to grieve the loss of a loved one for more than two weeks, then they have the chemical brain disease of major depressive disorder.

In other words, one is expected to not express too much distress if they are bullied and discriminated against for their gender non-conformity or ethnicity, to not express too much pain or confusion if one's parent is also one's attacker or sexual seducer, and to not be sad for more than 14 days if your best friend dies or you lose your child. If you show too much pain, need too much from others, struggle to overcome your anger and resentment, or do not rejoin society and contribute to the workforce quick enough, you might be considered to be mentally ill and in need of expert treatments, possibly for life.

WHERE STIGMA BEGINS

Personally, I don't think that these labels are ever appropriate. I think that people talk in circles about the "stigma of mental illness" while we know that when you stop medicalizing people's experiences and look at what happened in that person's life and how these "symptoms" are serving them, that that's when you have a real chance to help them out. P1

Most of us are overwhelmed by the shame and the stigma and the terror that we'll never get jobs or that people might think that we are idiots. That stuff causes enormous harm and suffering. P5

That's what DBT is associated with: borderline/bitch. It's therapy for the bitches, basically. So, there's the stigma that comes with that, and it's sad because it can be really effective if there are good clinicians in charge who see past the bitch label. P13

Even without the societal, ideological, and scientific problems with diagnoses, there are still those who claim that such a framework helps individuals to be taken seriously, assists them in having their pain and suffering recognized and empathized with, and challenges the tendency to blame individuals for their problems. Someone who is suffering is no longer chastised for not being able to "just snap out of it" and pain is recognized as "real". But at what cost?

Once diagnosed, a person's sense of self and reality are altered, sometimes permanently (Knight, Wykes, & Hayward, 2003; Leete, 1989). For those who have experienced abuse, bullying, discrimination, or oppression, a diagnosis effectively implies that the problem is within the individual, often reinforcing dynamics of denial, gaslighting, and scapegoating. For many, this labeling has the effect of increasing feelings of being unacceptable, different, defective, "dirty", powerless, and subject to the demands of powerful others (Chernomas, Clarke, & Chisholm, 2000; Knight et al., 2003). The more one agrees with a medicalized, diagnostic framework, the greater the depression, the greater the likelihood for suicide, and the less one believes he or she has agency for his or her behaviors (Crumlish et al., 2005; Easter, 2012; Seeman, 2009). In addition, individuals who internalize this illness model tend to have worse functioning (Carter, Read, Pyle, & Morrison, 2016; Deacon, 2013; Gammell & Stoppard, 1999), are less likely to experience subjective recovery due to increased hopelessness and lower self-esteem (Vass, Sitko, West, & Bentall, 2017), and are less likely to seek help (Clement et al., 2015).

Aside from this internalized sense of defectiveness, practitioners, too, tend to have increased prejudice and negative attitudes toward individuals seeking help when they adhere to this illness paradigm. Those who believe that diagnoses are important and a central part of effective treatment tend to be less empathic, less effective, and more judgmental (Deacon, 2013; Read, Haslam, Sayce, & Davies, 2006). A biogenetic conceptualization of individuals also leads clinicians to perceive their patients as less human, and, in turn, they are more likely to support acts of control or coercion, such as physical restraint (Pavon & Vaes, 2017).

The public, too, has been shown to react to the illness model of emotional distress with disdain and increased negative attitudes. In general, the public tends to react to individuals with severe mental illness diagnoses with fear and a desire to exclude such individuals from society, paternalism and the belief that such individuals cannot make their own life decisions, and an impression that persons with these diagnoses are like children (Brockington, Hall, Levings, & Murphy, 1993; Read et al., 2006; Rüsch, Todd, Bodenhausen, & Corrigan, 2010). Interestingly, people diagnosed with mental illness are perceived as actually being *more* responsible for their problems than are those whose struggles are contextualized within their life circumstances (Corrigan et al., 2000; Read & Harre, 2001). Overall, there is strong agreement, as seen through several studies on stigma, that the mental illness paradigm and focus on biological disease has not worked and may actually have made things worse (see Malla, Joober, & Garcia, 2015 for an overview). When a socially constructed difference is created (i.e., diagnoses and mental illness), this inevitably becomes a source for prejudice and discrimination (e.g., Liegghio, 2016), and the evidence shows that diagnoses have become fodder for just that.

On the other hand, higher proportions of healing are found in those societies that do not adopt the Western model of illness (e.g., Jaaskelainen et al., 2013). Additionally, validation, empathy, a solid therapeutic relationship, empowerment, hope, and direct work with trauma-related and so-called psychotic-related phenomena from a psychosocial framework may be sufficient without ever needing to resort to utilizing hypothetical, medically based diagnoses (see Thomas & Longden, 2013 for a discussion).

NOTES

1. See, for example, O'Brien (2016), McDonald (1997), and Pihlajamaki (2000), for analyses and reviews of practices common during the sixteenth and seventeenth centuries. Most reviews of the time view these practices as highly biased, stemming from fear and attempts to control the chaos and suffering in life through the prevailing ideology of the time (i.e., Christianity). These reviews, and many others, highlight how the certainty of the professionals of the time was an illusion and resulted in the torture and death of countless innocent victims. See, specifically, Pihlajamaki, for an analysis of how professionalism and a "scientification" of the procedures involved helped explain why these witchcraft trials and ordeals were so common in countries whose values aligned with science and professional stature.
2. In almost every psychological and/or neurological battery ordered, an IQ test will be included to examine for "cognitive deficits" or "areas of weakness" that are purported to be associated with particular diagnostic categories. The subtest titled "Information" specifically requires individuals to know random facts, for example, "Who is Martin Luther King, Jr.?" or "Who authored *Tom Sawyer*?" The subtest regarding Comprehension requires individuals to have a particularly narrow view of things like keeping money in a bank or putting envelopes in the mail. While common, these are not universal, nor, certainly, evidence of anything other than someone's Westernized educated culture and conforming attitude. In addition to this more formal test, if a person speaks in convoluted or confusing ways, they may be said to "have a thought disorder", which is presumed to be evidence of brain dysfunction or disease rather than, perhaps, confusion due to trauma or prolonged stress, drugs (prescribed or not), or just mere lack of desire to communicate in proscribed ways.
3. See, for example, Kinderman et al. (2017) and Pilgrim (2014) for recent analyses and reviews of the history of the politics controlling the development of and subsequent changes to the *DSM*, and the uproar in response to the latest version. See also Caplan (1995) and Ross (2008) for critical insiders' reflections on the development of diagnoses and the *DSM*. All offer rich information on the details of this process throughout the years, a glimpse behind the scenes of what really goes on, and analyses of how political and financial agendas in accordance with societal needs appear to guide the process rather than true science.
4. There are numerous analyses of the history of many of these drugs, the political and even corrupt practices of pharmaceutical companies and their representative researchers and ghostwriters, and the lack of long-term effectiveness, specificity, and harm associated with psychotropic drugs. For instance, see Healy (2012) for a detailed account of how the pharma-centric

system of care has decreased the ability to actually care, and how corruption and greed have resulted in millions taking unnecessary and even harmful drugs that are sold as "life-savers". See also Moncrieff (2013) for a critical historical analysis of neuroleptic drugs, the story that developed from one of dangerous and largely ineffective drugs to "magic bullets" that are antipsychotics, and the current epidemic of prescribing. Additional evaluative narratives that highlight a broader truth than typically spread regarding these drugs and the medicalization of human suffering include, but certainly is not limited to Kirk, Gomory, and Cohen (2013); Olfman and Robbins (2012); Rapley, Moncrieff, and Dillon (2011); and Whitaker (2010).

5. I myself am a clinical psychologist operating under this paradigm. Most of the people I work with pay through insurance. Insurance companies only reimburse for medical problems—in fact, if they determine that a person's issues are spiritual, existential, or otherwise non-medical, I will stop getting paid. I, like all of my colleagues, have a vested interest in maintaining this setup seeing as how I cannot pay rent without it. Further, I live in New York City where the population of therapists is rivaled only by that, perhaps, of actors, finance professionals, and rats. One must be able to stand out, and the only way to do this is through having a "specialty". Without diagnoses, what would we specialize in? I have lost not a few potential clients as a result of my refusal to pretend that I specialize in anything other than supporting people in better understanding and working through their human suffering. See also Whitaker and Cosgrove (2015) for an academic thesis on how these guild interests fuel corruption and promotion of the status quo.

6. In society, in general, women frequently get blamed for putting themselves in a position that enticed a rapist or allowed sexual abuse or rape to occur (e.g., Deming, Covan, Swan, & Billings, 2013). It has also been asserted that prolonged distress after experiences such as sexual abuse is the result of problematic ways of thinking or an innate temperament (e.g., Hankin & Abramson, 2001) rather than this being an understandable result of extraordinary circumstances. What if, instead of words like "personality disorder" or "schizophrenia" or "dissociative disorder", we started classifying people as having "sexual abuse reaction syndrome"? How would this change the way we interact with and care for such individuals?

7. See, for instance, Levine (2011), for an exploration of how democracy, economic injustices, and elitism have contributed to the silencing and powerlessness of individuals who either do not or cannot conform. Bruce Levine has written numerous articles, blogs, and books about the pathologizing and diagnosing of anti-authoritarians and non-conformists. He also offers potential solutions for uniting and changing the status quo. See brucelevine.net.

REFERENCES

Abel, K. M., Drake, R., & Goldstein, J. M. (2010). Sex differences in schizophrenia. *International Review of Psychiatry, 22*(5), 417–428.

Addis, M. E., & Mahalik, J. R. (2003). Men, masculinity, and the contexts of help seeking. *American Psychologist, 58*, 5–14.

Altshuler, L. L., Kupka, R. W., Hellemann, G., Frye, M. A., Sugar, C. A., McElroy, S. L., … Suppes, T. (2010). Gender and depressive symptoms in 711 patients with bipolar disorder evaluated prospectively in the Stanley Foundation Bipolar Treatment Outcome Network. *American Journal of Psychiatry, 167*(6), 708–715.

American Psychiatric Association. (2013). *Diagnostic and statistical manual of mental disorders: DSM-5.* Washington, DC: American Psychiatric Association.

Barnes, A. (2008). Race and hospital diagnoses of schizophrenia and mood disorders. *Social Work, 53*(1), 77–83.

Barnes, A. (2013). Race and schizophrenia in four types of hospitals. *Journal of Black Studies, 44*(6), 665–681.

Barstow, A. L. (1988). On studying witchcraft as women's history: A historiography of the European witch persecutions. *Journal of Feminist Studies in Religion, 4*(2), 7–19.

Bentall, R. P. (2003). *Madness explained: Psychosis and human nature.* London: Penguin.

Blanchard, M., & Farber, B. A. (2016). Lying in psychotherapy: Why and what clients don't tell their therapist about therapy and their relationship. *Counselling Psychology Quarterly, 29*(1), 90–112.

Brand, B. L., Myrick, A., Loewenstein, R. J., Classen, C. C., Lanius, R., McNary, S. W., … Putnam, F. W. (2012). A survey of practices and recommended treatment interventions among expert therapists treating patients with dissociative identity disorder and dissociative disorder not otherwise specified. *Psychological Trauma: Theory, Research, Practice, and Policy, 4*(5), 490–500.

British Psychological Society. (2013). Division of Clinical Psychology position statement on the classification of behaviour and experience in relation to functional psychiatric diagnoses: Time for a paradigm shift. Retrieved from http:// dxrevisionwatch.files.wordpress.com/2013/05/position-statement-on-diagnosis-master-doc.pdf

Brockington, I. F., Hall, P., Levings, J., & Murphy, C. (1993). The community's tolerance of the mentally ill. *British Journal of Psychiatry, 162*, 93–99.

Brown, L. S. (1992). A feminist critique of the personality disorders. In L. S. Brown & M. Ballou (Eds.), *Personality and psychopathology: Feminist reappraisals* (pp. 206–228). New York: Guilford.

Burstow, B. (2017). Psychiatric drugging of children and youth as a form of child abuse: Not a radical proposition. *Ethical Human Psychology and Psychiatry, 19*(1), 65–76.

Bussey, K., & Bandura, A. (1999). Social cognitive theory of gender development and differentiation. *Psychological Review, 106,* 676–713.

Bynum, B. (2000). Discarded diagnoses. *The Lancet, 356*(9241), 1615.

Caplan, P. J. (1995). *They say you're crazy: How the world's most powerful psychiatrists decide who's normal.* Reading, MA: Addison-Wesley.

Carlson, E. B., Dalenberg, C., & McDade-Montez, E. (2012). Dissociation in posttraumatic stress disorder Part 1: Definitions and review of research. *Psychological Trauma: Theory, Research, Practice, and Policy, 4*(5), 479–489.

Carlson, E. B., & Putnam, F. W. (1993). An update on the dissociative experiences scale. *Dissociation, 6,* 16–27.

Carter, L., Read, J., Pyle, M., & Morrison, A. P. (2016). The impact of causal explanations on outcome in people experiencing psychosis: A systematic review. *Clinical Psychology & Psychotherapy.* https://doi.org/10.1002/cpp.2002

Cassiman, S. A. (2008). Of witches, welfare queens, and the disaster named poverty: The search for a counter-narrative. *Journal of Poverty, 10*(4), 51–66.

Chernomas, W. M., Clarke, D. E., & Chisholm, F. A. (2000). Perspectives of women living with schizophrenia. *Psychiatric Services, 51*(12), 1517–1521.

Chien, W. T., & Thompson, D. (2014). Effects of a mindfulness-based psycho-education programme for Chines patients with schizophrenia: 2-year follow-up. *British Journal of Psychiatry, 205*(1), 52–59.

Cicchetti, D. (1994). Guidelines, criteria, and rules of thumb for evaluating normed and standardized assessment instruments in psychology. *Psychological Assessment, 6*(4), 284–290.

Clement, S., Schauman, O., Graham, T., Maggioni, F., Evans-Lacko, S., Bezborodovs, N., ... Thornicroft, G. (2015). What is the impact of mental health-related stigma on help-seeking? A systematic review of quantitative and qualitative studies. *Psychological Medicine, 45*(1), 11–27.

Coleman, K. J., Stewart, C., Waitzfelder, B. E., Zeber, J. E., Morales, L. S., Ahmed, A. T., ... Simon, G. E. (2016). Racial-ethnic differences in psychiatric diagnoses and treatment across 11 health care systems in the mental health research network. *Psychiatric Services, 67*(7), 749–757.

Cook, E. P., Warnke, M., & Dupuy, P. (1993). Gender bias and the DSM-III-R. *Counselor Education and Supervision, 32*(4), 311–322.

Corrigan, P. W., River, L. P., Lundin, R. K., Wasowski, K. U., Campion, J., Mathisen, J., ... Kubiak, M. A. (2000). Stigmatizing attributions about mental illness. *Journal of Community Psychology, 28*(1), 91–102.

Cotton, S. M., Lambert, M., Schimmelmann, B. G., Foley, D. L., Morley, K. L., McGorry, P. D., & Conus, P. (2009). Gender differences in premorbid, entry, treatment, and outcome characteristics in a treated epidemiological sample of 661 patients with first episode psychosis. *Schizophrenia Research, 114,* 17–24.

Coughlan, H., & Cannon, M. (2017). Does childhood trauma play a role in the aetiology of psychosis? A review of recent evidence. *BJPsych Advances, 23*(5), 307–315.

THE ILLNESS INQUISITION   87

Crowell, S. E., Beauchaine, T. P., & Linehan, M. M. (2009). A biosocial developmental model of borderline personality: Elaborating and extending Linehan's theory. *Psychological Bulletin, 135*(3), 495–510.

Crumlish, N., Whitty, P., Kamali, M., Clarke, M., Browne, S., McTique, O., ... O'Callaghan, E. (2005). Early insight predicts depression and attempted suicide after 4 years in first-episode schizophrenia and schizophreniform disorder. *Acta Psychiatrica Scandinavica, 112*(6), 449–455.

Dalenberg, C., & Carlson, E. B. (2012). Dissociation in posttraumatic stress disorder part II: How theoretical models fit the empirical evidence and recommendations for modifying the diagnostic criteria for PTSD. *Psychological Trauma: Theory, Research, Practice, and Policy, 4*(6), 551–559.

De Fruyt, J., & Demyttenaere, K. (2004). Rapid tranquilization: New approaches in the emergency treatment of behavioral disturbances. *European Psychiatry, 19*(5), 243–249.

Deacon, B. J. (2013). The biomedical model of mental disorder: A critical analysis of its validity, utility, and effects on psychotherapy research. *Clinical Psychology Review, 33*, 846–861.

Deming, M. E., Covan, E. K., Swan, S. C., & Billings, D. L. (2013). Exploring rape myths, gendered norms, group processing, and the social context of rape among college women: A qualitative analysis. *Violence Against Women, 19*(4), 465–485.

Desai, B., Summers, A., & Bunker, N. (2013). Borderline traits as a risk factor for adverse outcomes in psychosis. *Psychosis, 5*(2), 200–202.

Dubin, W. R., & Feld, J. A. (1989). Rapid tranquilization of the violent patient. *The American Journal of Emergency Medicine, 7*(3), 313–320.

Easter, M. M. (2012). "Not all my fault": Genetics, stigma, and personal responsibility for women with eating disorders. *Social Science & Medicine, 75*(8), 1408–1416. https://doi.org/10.1016/j.socscimed.2012.05.042

Ellason, J. W., Ross, C. A., & Fuchs, D. L. (1996). Lifetime axis I and II comorbidity and childhood trauma history in dissociative identity disorder. *Psychiatry, 59*, 255–266.

Erlandsson, S., & Punzi, E. (2016). Challenging the ADHD consensus. *International Journal of Qualitative Studies on Health and Well-Being, 11*. https://doi.org/10.3402/qhw.v11.31124

Fabrega, H. (1996). Cultural and historical foundations of psychiatric diagnosis. In J. E. Mezzich, A. Kleinman, H. Fabrega, & D. L. Parron (Eds.), *Culture and psychiatric diagnosis: A DSM-IV perspective* (pp. 3–14). Washington, DC: American Psychiatric Press.

Feisthamel, K. P., & Schwartz, R. C. (2009). Differences in mental health counselors' diagnoses based on client race: An investigation of adjustment, childhood, and substance-related disorders. *Journal of Mental Health Counseling, 31*(10), 47–59.

Fleischhacker, W. W., Kane, J. M., Geier, J., Karayal, O., Kolluri, S., Eng, S. M., ... Strom, B. L. (2014). Completed and attempted suicides among 18,154 subjects with schizophrenia included in a large simple trial. *Journal of Clinical Psychiatry, 75*(3), e184–e190. https://doi.org/10.4088/JCP.13m08563

Foote, B., & Park, J. (2008). Dissociative identity disorder and schizophrenia: Differential diagnosis and theoretical issues. *Current Psychiatry Reports, 10*(3), 217–222.

Foulks, E. F. (2004). Cultural variables in psychiatry. *Psychiatric Times, 21*, 28–29.

Frances, A. (2016). A report card on the utility of psychiatric diagnosis. *World Psychiatry, 15*, 32–33.

Freeman, D., & Garety, P. A. (2003). Connecting neurosis and psychosis: The direct influence of emotion on delusions and hallucinations. *Behavior Research and Therapy, 41*(8), 923–947.

Frueh, B. C., Grubaugh, A. L., Cusack, K. J., Kimble, M. O., Elhai, J. D., & Knapp, R. G. (2009). Exposure-based cognitive behavioral treatment of PTSD in adults with schizophrenia or schizoaffective disorder. *Journal of Anxiety Disorders, 23*(5), 665–675.

Gammell, D. J., & Stoppard, J. M. (1999). Women's experiences of treatment of depression: Medicalization or empowerment? *Canadian Psychology, 40*(2), 112–128.

Gillig, P. M. (2009). Dissociative identity disorder: A controversial diagnosis. *Psychiatry (Edgmont), 6*(3), 24–29.

Goldstein, J. M. (1995). The impact of gender on understanding the epidemiology of schizophrenia. In M. V. Seeman (Ed.), *Gender and psychopathology* (pp. 159–199). Washington, DC: American Psychiatric Press.

Greenberg, G. (2010). *Manufacturing depression: The secret history of a modern disease.* New York: Simon & Schuster.

Gunderson, J. G., Weinberg, I., Daversa, M. T., Kueppenbender, K. D., Zanarini, M. C., Shea, M. T., ... Dyck, I. (2006). Descriptive and longitudinal observations on the relationship of borderline personality disorder and bipolar disorder. *American Journal of Psychiatry, 163*, 1173–1178.

Hankin, B. J., & Abramson, L. Y. (2001). Development of gender differences in depression: An elaborated cognitive vulnerability-transactional stress theory. *Psychological Bulletin, 127*(6), 773–796.

Hare-Mustin, R. T., & Marecek, J. (1997). Abnormal and clinical psychology: The politics of madness. In D. Fox & I. Prilleltensky (Eds.), *Critical psychology: An introduction.* London: SAGE.

Hartung, C. M., & Widiger, T. A. (1998). Gender differences in the diagnosis of mental disorders: Conclusions and controversies of the DSM-IV. *Psychological Bulletin, 123*(3), 260–278.

Healy, D. (2012). *Pharmageddon.* Los Angeles, CA: University of California Press.

Hornstein, G. A. (2013). Whose account matters? A challenge to feminist psychologists. *Feminism & Psychology, 23*, 29–40.

Howell, E. (2008). From hysteria to chronic relational trauma disorder: The history of borderline personality disorder and its links with dissociation and psychosis. In A. Moskowitz, I. Schafer, & M. J. Dorahy (Eds.), *Psychosis, trauma and dissociation: Emerging perspectives on severe psychopathology* (pp. 105–115). West Sussex: Wiley & Sons, Ltd.

Hurst, S. A., & Genest, M. (1995). Cognitive-behavioural therapy with a feminist orientation: A perspective for therapy with depressed women. *Canadian Psychology, 36*(3), 236–257.

Jaaskelainen, E., Juola, P., Hirvonen, N., McGrath, J. J., Saha, S., Isohanni, M., … Miettunen, J. (2013). A systematic review and meta-analysis of recovery in schizophrenia. *Schizophrenia Bulletin, 39*(6), 1296–1306.

Jablensky, A., & Sartorius, N. (2008). What did the WHO studies really find? *Schizophrenia Bulletin, 34*(2), 253–255.

Jackson, L. (1995). Witches, wives and mothers: Witchcraft persecution and women's confessions in seventeenth-century England. *Women's History Review, 4*(1), 63–84.

Jacobson, N. C., & Newman, M. G. (2017). Anxiety and depression as bidirectional risk factors for one another: A meta-analysis of longitudinal studies. *Psychological Bulletin, 143*(11), 1155–1200.

Johnstone, L. (2014). *A straight talking introduction to psychiatric diagnosis.* Monmouth: PCCS Books Ltd.

Jost, J. T., Hawkins, C. B., Nosek, B. A., Hennes, E. P., Stern, C., Gosling, S. D., & Graham, J. (2013). Belief in a just God (and a just society): A system justification perspective on religious ideology. *Journal of Theoretical and Philosophical Psychology, 34*(1), 56–81.

Kelleher, I., & Cannon, M. (2016). Putting psychosis in its place. [Editorial]. *American Journal of Psychiatry, 173*(10), 951–952.

Kernberg, O. F. (1975). *Borderline conditions and pathological narcissism.* Northvale, NJ: Jason Aronson.

Kinderman, P., Allsopp, K., & Cooke, A. (2017). Responses to the publication of the american psychiatric association's DSM-5. *Journal of Humanistic Psychology, 57*(6), 625–649. https://doi.org/10.1177/0022167817698262

Kingdon, D. G., Ashcroft, K., Bhandari, B., Gleeson, S., Warikoo, N., Symons, M., … Mehta, R. (2010). Schizophrenia and borderline personality disorder: Similarities and differences in the experience of auditory hallucinations, paranoia, and childhood trauma. *Journal of Nervous and Mental Disease, 198*(6), 399–403.

Kirk, S. A., Gomory, T., & Cohen, D. (2013). *Mad science: Psychiatric coercion, diagnosis, and drugs.* New Brunswick, NJ: Transaction Publishers.

Kirkbride, J. B., Hameed, Y., Ioannidis, K., Ankireddypalli, G., Crane, C. M., Nasir, M., ... Jones, P. B. (2017). Ethnic minority status, age-at-immigration and psychosis risk in rural environments: Evidence form the SEPEA Study. *Schizophrenia Bulletin.* https://doi.org/10.1093/schbul/sbx010

Kirsch, I., Deacon, B. J., Huedo-Medina, T. B., Scoboria, A., Moore, T. J., & Johnson, B. T. (2008). Initial severity and antidepressant benefits: A meta-analysis of data submitted to the Food and Drug Administration. *PLoS Medicine, 5*(2), e45.

Knight, M. T. D., Wykes, T., & Hayward, P. (2003). "People don't understand": An investigation of stigma in schizophrenia using Interpretative Phenomenological Analysis (IPA). *Journal of Mental Health, 12*(3), 209–222.

Kraemer, H. C., Kupfer, D. J., Clarke, D. E., Narrow, W. E., & Regier, D. A. (2012). DSM-5: How reliable is reliable enough? *American Journal of Psychiatry, 169,* 13–15.

Kupfer, D. J. (2013). News release: Chair of DSM-5 task force discusses future of mental health research. *American Psychiatric Association.* Retrieved from www.psychiatry.org

Lakhan, S. E., & Kirchgessner, A. (2012). Prescription stimulants in individuals with and without attention deficit hyperactivity disorder: Misuse, cognitive impact, and adverse effects. *Brain and Behavior, 2*(5), 661–677.

Lanius, R., Brand, B. L., Vermetten, E., Frewen, P. A., & Spiegel, D. (2012). The dissociative subtype of posttraumatic stress disorder: Rationale, clinical and neurobiological evidence, and implications. *Depression and Anxiety, 29,* 701–708.

Lanius, R., Vermetten, E., Loewenstein, R. J., Brand, B. L., Schmahl, C., Bremner, J. D., & Spiegel, D. (2010). Emotion modulation in PTSD: Clinical and neurobiological evidence for a dissociative subtype. *The American Journal of Psychiatry, 167*(6), 640–647.

Lauer, J., Black, D. W., & Keen, P. (1993). Multiple personality disorder and borderline personality disorder: Distinct entities or variations on a common theme? *Annals of Clinical Psychiatry, 5,* 129–134.

Leete, E. (1989). How I perceive and manage my illness. *Schizophrenia Bulletin, 15,* 197–200.

Levine, B. E. (2011). *Get up, stand up: Uniting populists, energizing the defeated, and battling the corporate elite.* White River Junction, VT: Chelsea Green Pub.

Liegghio, M. (2016). Too young to be mad: Disabling encounters with 'normal' from the perspectives of psychiatrized youth. *Intersectionalities: A Global Journal of Social Work Analysis, Research, Polity, and Practice, 5*(3), 110–129.

Liotti, G., & Gumley, A. (2008). An attachment perspective on schizophrenia: The role of disorganized attachment, dissociation and mentalization. In A. Moskowitz, I. Schafer, & M. J. Dorahy (Eds.), *Psychosis, trauma and disso-*

ciation: Emerging perspectives on severe psychopathology (pp. 117–133). West Sussex: John Wiley & Sons, Ltd.

Malla, A., Joober, R., & Garcia, A. (2015). "Mental illness is like any other medical illness": A critical examination of the statement and its impact on patient care and society. *Journal of Psychiatry & Neuroscience: JPN, 40*(3), 147–150. https://doi.org/10.1503/jpn.150099

Marecek, J. (2006). Social suffering, gender, and women's depression. In C. L. Keyes & S. H. Goodman (Eds.), *Women and depression: A handbook for the social, behavioral, and biomedical sciences* (pp. 283–308). Cambridge: Cambridge University Press.

Mayes, R., & Horwitz, A. V. (2005). DSM-III and the revolution in the classification of mental illness. *Journal of the History of the Behavioral Sciences, 41*(3), 249–267.

McDonald, S. W. (1997). The Devil's mark and the witch-prickers of Scotland. *Journal of the Royal Society of Medicine, 90,* 507–511.

McGilloway, A., Hall, R. E., Lee, T., & Bhui, K. S. (2010). A systematic review of personality disorder, race and ethnicity: Prevalence, aetiology and treatment. *BMC Psychiatry, 10,* 33. https://doi.org/10.1186/1471-244X-10-33

McLean, B. (2001, August). A bitter pill Prozac made Eli Lilly. Then along came a feisty generic maker called Barr Labs. Their battle gives new meaning to the term "drug war." *Fortune Magazine.* Retrieved from http://archive.fortune.com/magazines/fortune/fortune_archive/2001/08/13/308077/index.htm

McWilliams, N. (2015). More simply human: On the universality of madness. *Psychosis, 7*(1), 63–71.

Mehl-Madrona, L., Jul, E., & Mainguy, B. (2014). Results of a transpersonal, narrative, and phenomenological psychotherapy for psychosis. *International Journal of Transpersonal Studies, 33*(1), 57–76.

Metzl, J. M. (2010). *The protest psychosis: How schizophrenia became a black disease.* Boston, MA: Beacon Press.

Middleton, W., Dorahy, M. J., & Moskowitz, A. (2008). Historical conceptions of dissociation and psychosis: Nineteenth and early twentieth century perspectives on severe psychopathology. In A. Moskowitz, I. Schafer, & M. J. Dorahy (Eds.), *Psychosis, trauma, and dissociation: Emerging perspectives on severe psychopathology.* Wiley-Blackwell: West Sussex.

Moncrieff, J. (2008). *The myth of the chemical cure: A critique of psychiatric drug treatment.* Basingstoke: Palgrave Macmillan.

Moncrieff, J. (2013). *The bitterest pills: The troubling story of antipsychotic drugs.* Basingstoke: Palgrave Macmillan.

Morrison, A. P. (2001). The interpretation of intrusions in psychosis: An integrative cognitive approach to psychotic symptoms. *Behavioural & Cognitive Psychotherapy, 29,* 257–276.

Morrison, A. P., Frame, L., & Larkin, W. (2003). Relationships between trauma and psychosis: A review and integration. *British Journal of Clinical Psychology*, *42*, 331–353.

Morrison, A. P., Hutton, P., Shiers, D., & Turkington, D. (2012). Antipsychotics: Is it time to introduce patient choice? *British Journal of Psychiatry*, *201*, 83–84.

Moskowitz, A. (2008). Association and dissociation in the historical concept of schizophrenia. In A. Moskowitz, I. Schafer, & M. J. Dorahy (Eds.), *Psychosis, trauma and dissociation: Emerging perspectives on severe psychopathology* (pp. 35–49). West Sussex: John Wiley & Sons, Ltd.

Moskowitz, A., Read, J., Farrelly, S., Rudegeair, T., & Williams, O. (2009). Are psychotic symptoms traumatic in origin and dissociative in kind? In P. F. Dell & J. A. O'Neil (Eds.), *Dissociation and the dissociative disorders: DSM-V and beyond* (pp. 521–534). New York: Routledge.

Neighbors, H. W., Jackson, J. S., Campbell, L., & Williams, D. (1989). The influence of racial factors on psychiatric diagnosis: A review and suggestions for research. *Community Mental Health Journal*, *25*(4), 301–311.

Neighbors, H. W., Trierweiler, S. J., Ford, B. C., & Muroff, J. R. (2003). Racial differences in DSM diagnosis using a semi-structured instrument: The importance of clinical judgment in the diagnosis of African Americans. *Journal of Health and Social Behavior*, *44*(3), 237–256.

Nguyen, L., Huang, L. N., Arganza, G. F., & Liao, Q. (2007). The influence of race and ethnicity on psychiatric diagnoses and clinical characteristics of children and adolescents in children's services. *Cultural Diversity and Ethnic Minority Psychology*, *13*, 18–25.

O'Brien, S. I. (2016). The discovery of witches: Matthew Hopkins's defense of his witch-hunting methods. *Preternature*, *5*(1), 29–58.

O'Neill, J. (1986). The medicalization of social control. *Canadian Review of Sociology*, *23*(3), 350–364.

Olfman, S., & Robbins, B. D. (Eds.). (2012). *Drugging our children: How profiteers are pushing antipsychotics on our youngest, and what we can do to stop it*. Santa Barbara, CA: Praeger.

Owen, M. J. (2014). New approaches to psychiatric diagnostic classification. *Neuron*, *84*(3), 564–571.

Paris, J., Brown, R., & Nowlis, D. (2001). A 27-year follow-up of patients with borderline personality disorder. *Comprehensive Psychiatry*, *42*, 482–487.

Parker, G. (2014). Is borderline personality disorder a mood disorder? *The British Journal of Psychiatry*, *204*(4), 252–253. https://doi.org/10.1192/bjp.bp.113.136580

Parks, J., Hillard, J. R., & Gillig, P. M. (1989). Jane and John Doe in the psychiatric emergency service. *The Psychiatric Quarterly*, *60*(4), 297–302.

Pavon, G., & Vaes, J. (2017). Bio-genetic vs. psycho-environmental conceptions of schizophrenia and their role in perceiving patients in human terms. *Psychosis*, *9*(3), 245–253.

Penfold, S., & Walker, G. (1984). *Women and the psychiatric paradox*. Milton Keynes: Open University Press.

Pies, R. W. (2011, July). Psychiatry's new brain-mind and the legend of the "chemical imbalance". *Psychiatric Times*. Retrieved from http://www.psychiatrictimes.com/blogs/psychiatry-new-brain-mind-and-legend-chemical-imbalance

Pihlajamaki, H. (2000). 'Swimming the witch, pricking for the Devil's mark': Ordeals in the early modern witchcraft trials. *The Journal of Legal History, 21*(2), 35–58.

Pilgrim, D. (2014). Historical resonances of the DSM-5 dispute: American exceptionalism or Eurocentrism? *History of the Human Sciences, 27*(2), 97–117. https://doi.org/10.1177/0952695114527998

Pokos, V., & Castle, D. J. (2006). Prevalence of comorbid anxiety disorders in schizophrenia spectrum disorders: A literature review. *Current Psychiatry Reviews, 2*(3), 285–307. https://doi.org/10.2174/157340006778018193

Rapley, M., Moncrieff, J., & Dillon, J. (Eds.). (2011). *De-medicalizing misery: Psychiatry, psychology and the human condition*. Basingstoke: Palgrave Macmillan.

Read, J. (1997). Child abuse and psychosis: A literature review and implications for professionals. *Professional Psychology: Research and Practice, 28*(5), 448–456.

Read, J., & Harre, N. (2001). The role of biological and genetic causal beliefs in the stigmatization of 'mental patients'. *Journal of Mental Health, 10*(2), 223–235.

Read, J., Haslam, N., Sayce, L., & Davies, E. (2006). Prejudice and schizophrenia: A review of the 'mental illness is an illness like any other' approach. *Acta Psychiatrica Scandinavica, 114*(5), 303–318.

Read, J., van Os, J., Morrison, A. P., & Ross, C. A. (2005). Childhood trauma, psychosis, and schizophrenia: A literature review with theoretical and clinical implications. *Acta Psychiatrica Scandinavica, 112*, 330–350.

Regier, D. A., Narrow, W. E., Clarke, D. E., Kraemer, H. C., Kuramoto, S. J., Kuhl, E. A., & Kupfer, D. J. (2013). DSM-5 field trials in the United States and Canada, Part II: Test-retest reliability of selected categorical diagnoses. *American Journal of Psychiatry, 170*, 59–70.

Ross, C. A. (2008). *The great psychiatry scam: One shrink's personal journey*. Richardson, TX: Manitou Communications, Inc.

Ross, C. A., & Keyes, B. (2004). Dissociation and schizophrenia. *Journal of Trauma & Dissociation, 5*(3), 69–83.

Rüsch, N., Todd, A. R., Bodenhausen, G. V., & Corrigan, P. W. (2010). Biogenetic models of psychopathology, implicit guilt, and mental illness stigma. *Psychiatry Research, 179*(3), 328–332. https://doi.org/10.1016/j.psychres.2009.09.010

Salokangas, R. K., Vaahtera, K., Pacriev, S., Sohlman, B., & Lehtinen, V. (2002). Gender differences in depressive symptoms: An artefact caused by measurement instruments. *Journal of Affective Disorders, 68*, 215–220.

Sansone, R. A., & Sansone, L. A. (2011). Gender patterns in borderline personality disorder. *Innovations in Clinical Neuroscience, 8*, 16–20.

Sar, V., Taycan, O., Bolat, N., Ozmen, M., Duran, A., Ozturk, E., & Ertem-Vehid, H. (2010). Childhood trauma and dissociation in schizophrenia. *Psychopathology, 43*(1), 33–40.

Saul, R. (2014). *ADHD does not exist: The truth about attention deficit and hyperactivity disorder.* New York: Harper Wave.

Schultz, W., & Hunter, N. (2016). Depression, chemical imbalances, and feminism. *Journal of Feminist Family Therapy, 28*(4), 159–173.

Seeman, M. V. (2009). Suicide among women with schizophrenia spectrum disorders. *American Journal of Psychiatry, 154*(12), 1641–1647.

Shaw, C., & Proctor, G. (2005). Women at the margins: A critique of the diagnosis of borderline personality disorder. *Feminism & Psychology, 15*(4), 483–490.

Smith, D. J., Muir, W. J., & Blackwood, D. H. R. (2004). Is borderline personality disorder part of the bipolar spectrum? *Harvard Review of Psychiatry, 12*, 133–139.

Smith, M. (2002). The flying phallus and the laughing inquisitor: Penis theft in the "Malleus Maleficarum". *Journal of Folklore Research, 39*(1), 85–117.

Stark, E., & Flitcraft, A. H. (1988). Women and children at risk: A feminist perspective on child abuse. *International Journal of Health Services, 18*, 97–118.

Stephens, W. (1998). Witches who steal penises: Impotence and illusion in *Malleus Maleficarum*. *Journal of Medieval and Early Modern Studies, 28*(3), 495–529.

Tasca, C., Rapetti, M., Carta, M. G., & Fadda, B. (2012). Women and hysteria in the history of mental health. *Clinical Practice & Epidemiology in Mental Health, 8*, 110–119.

Thomas, P., & Longden, E. (2013). Madness, childhood adversity and narrative psychiatry: Caring and the moral imagination. *Medical Humanities, 39*(2), 119–125.

Unger, R., & Crawford, M. (1992). *Women and gender: A feminist psychology.* Philadelphia, PA: Temple University Press.

Upthegrove, R., Marwaha, S., & Birchwood, M. (2017). Depression and schizophrenia: Cause, consequence, or trans-diagnostic issue? *Schizophrenia Bulletin, 43*(2), 240–244.

Vanheule, S. (2017). *Psychiatric diagnosis revisited – From DSM to clinical case formulation.* New York: Palgrave Macmillan.

Varese, F., Udachina, A., Myin-Germeys, I., Oorschot, M., & Bentall, R. P. (2011). The relationship between dissociation and auditory verbal hallucinations in the flow of daily life of patients with psychosis. *Psychosis, 3*(1), 14–28.

Vass, V., Sitko, K., West, S., & Bentall, R. P. (2017). How stigma gets under the skin: The role of stigma, self-stigma and self-esteem in subjective recovery from psychosis. *Psychosis, 9*(3), 235–244.

Vogel, M., Braungardt, T., Grabe, H. J., Schneider, W., & Klauer, T. (2013). Detachment, compartmentalization, and schizophrenia: Linking dissociation and psychosis by subtype. *Journal of Trauma & Dissociation, 14*, 273–287.

Wade, J. C. (1993). Institutional racism: An analysis of the mental health system. *American Journal of Orthopsychiatry, 63*(4), 536–544.

Wakefield, J. C. (2016). Against utility. *World Psychiatry, 15*, 33–35.

Wasserman, G. A., McReynolds, L. S., Ko, S. J., Katz, L. M., & Carpenter, J. R. (2005). Gender differences in psychiatric disorders at juvenile probation intake. *American Journal of Public Health, 95*, 131–137.

Watters, E. (2010). *Crazy like us.* New York: Free Press.

Whitaker, R. (2010). *Anatomy of an epidemic: Magic bullets, psychiatric drugs and the astonishing rise of mental illness.* New York: Broadway Paperbacks.

Whitaker, R., & Cosgrove, L. (2015). *Psychiatry under the influence; Institutional corruption, social injury, and prescriptions for reform.* New York: Palgrave Macmillan.

Widiger, T. A., & Spitzer, R. L. (1991). Sex bias in the diagnosis of personality disorders: Conceptual and methodological issues. *Clinical Psychology Review, 11*(1), 1–22.

Willhite, R. K., Niendam, T. A., Bearden, C. E., Zinberg, J., O'Brien, M. P., & Cannon, T. D. (2008). Gender differences in symptoms, functioning and social support in patients at ultra-high risk for developing a psychotic disorder. *Schizophrenia Research, 104*, 237–245.

Wilson, M. (1993). DSM-III and the transformation of American psychiatry: A history. *American Journal of Psychiatry, 150*(3), 399–410. https://doi.org/10.1176/ajp.150.3.399

Wolf, E. J., Miller, M. W., Reardon, A. F., Ryabchenko, K. A., Castillo, D., & Freund, R. (2012). A latent class analysis of dissociation and posttraumatic stress disorder: Evidence for a dissociative subtype. *Archives of General Psychiatry, 69*(7), 698–705.

Zhang, X. Y., Chen, D. C., Xiu, M. H., Yang, F. D., Haile, C. N., Kosten, T. A., & Kosten, R. R. (2012). Gender differences in never-medicated first-episode schizophrenia and medicated chronic schizophrenia patients. *Journal of Clinical Psychiatry, 73*(7), 1025–1033.

Zimmerman, M. (2015, July 24). Diagnosis of psychiatric disorders not as important as outcomes: Psychiatrist evaluates diagnostic practices. *Science Daily.* Retrieved from www.sciencedaily.com/releases/2015/07/150724082502.htm

Zipursky, R. B., Reilly, T. J., & Murray, R. M. (2013). The myth of schizophrenia as a progressive brain disease. *Schizophrenia Bulletin, 39*(6), 1363–1372.

CHAPTER 5

Suffering Is Human

A lot of [what is helpful in therapy] is about holding spaces, offering up
chances to reframe, normalizing the experience. P5

Despite what the religion of psychiatry tells us, even the most bizarre-
appearing mental and behavioral experiences are usually very human,
understandable, and even adaptive functions of the psyche. Although it is
taken for granted that an identifiable line exists between mental illness and
mental wellness, or sanity and insanity, this line is not, in fact, so solid and
clear. There is a continuum of human experience, and the development of
even some of the most seemingly fantastical phenomena can be seen as
completely normal and logical when placed within the context of one's life
history. All humans are prone to bouts of anxiety, depression, obsession,
strange beliefs, and superstition, especially when distressed and/or in fear.

Cross-national lifetime rates of suicidal ideation are around 9% to 13%,
with almost 3% of the population attempting suicide (Nock et al., 2008;
World Health Organization, n.d.), demonstrating the high prevalence and
large public health concern of despair and hopelessness (Crosby, Han,
Ortega, Parks, & Gfroerer, 2011). An even greater prevalence may be seen
among mental health professionals, with some evidence indicating that
more than half of those seeking a career in mental health have experienced
suicidal ideation in their lifetime (Hunter, 2015). Overall, more than a
quarter of the population across Europe and the United States meets criteria for a mental illness in a given year (World Health Organization, n.d.),

© The Author(s) 2018
N. Hunter, *Trauma and Madness in Mental Health Services*,
https://doi.org/10.1007/978-3-319-91752-8_5

and mental health problems account for a major portion of disability and public health concerns, especially among youth (Patel, Flisher, Hetrick, & McGorry, 2007). Most people, though, can understand and relate to depression, anxiety, and even suicidality; more severe and seemingly extreme experiences, however, seem too far beyond what most might experience, too atypical, and so, therefore, must be real mental illness. Right?

When people endure extreme experiences, such as child abuse, pervasive racism, marginalization and bullying among peers, living in poverty in a country or region of wealth, withstand highly toxic or dysfunctional family dynamics, or experience chronic stress during sensitive developmental periods, or a combination of any of the above, then the ways in which one expresses his or her distress tend to also become more extreme. People fall apart, parts of the self become cut off or depersonalized ("not-me"), inner voices become audible, the world becomes a dangerous place with villains perceived around every corner, strange beliefs become elaborate unrealistic systems of meaning-making, and aggression and suicidality live within. And, all of these psychic phenomena are exhibited across a range of populations, in differing combinations, and with a wide variety of associated dysfunction (or no dysfunction at all!).

If one moves away from the need for diagnostic nomenclature, it can become clear that consequences of early childhood trauma and adversity can manifest in a multitude of ways, perhaps based on temperamental variables (Liotti & Gumley, 2008), and on a continuum of severity. Using a trauma model (see Ross, 2007) may negate the need for diagnostic categories all together. However, this becomes difficult when beliefs are so entrenched and fixed, and phenomena such as multiple selves, dissociation, altered states of consciousness, fantastical belief systems, and extrasensory sensations such as voices are perceived as separate, abnormal, and bizarre experiences outside of everyday human experience. Yet, when looking more closely at these experiences, it becomes clear that all of these phenomena are interrelated, understandable facets of the universal human experience and almost always make sense within the context of any given individual's life circumstances.

Multiplicity Is Universal

There's a true self and there's an ego, or a false self, and everybody in the world has one. It doesn't matter if you're mentally ill or not. P10

DID or Multiple Personality Disorder

The doctor, the physician I went to to get the referral basically said to me "Well that's really rare so I doubt you have that". Which was really frustrating to me because, and I said to him, I said "Well, ya know, by the very nature of it being rare somebody has to have it. So, why couldn't I?". P3

Then she came out and said "Well, while I was in college, they told me that [alters] don't exist ... That's what I was told, and that only idiots think that they do". And, she had gone to college, like, maybe 10 years ago, she got her PhD in counseling I think, so that was pretty weird. She said "I thought for sure that they didn't exist until I met you". P4

The basis of the diagnosis of DID, and also the common subject of controversy and entertainment, is the idea of an individual having multiple selves or personalities that are distinct. People experiencing extreme dissociative states have been portrayed in numerous movies and television shows, such as: *The Three Faces of Eve, Sybil, Voices Within: The Lives of Truddi Chase, I Never Promised you a Rose Garden, Raising Cain, Shutter Island, Fight Club, United States of Tara, Split, Black Swan,* and *Mr. Robot.* One may be led to believe from these depictions that DID is a rare and flagrant disorder which can be easily identified by expert doctors who communicate effortlessly with different people in one body. And, with these improbable presentations, detractors within and out of the mental health field have persevered with cries of foul play and deceit.

Two books have been published regarding the case of Sybil, which was based on a true story, that make accusations that DID is a socially constructed disorder that is iatrogenically produced and reinforced by unethical and irresponsible therapeutic practices (Nathan, 2011; Rieber, 2006). Of course, all diagnoses are socially constructed categories and none are entirely iatrogenic or non-iatrogenic (Ross, 1990). These authors, however, specifically refer to the practice of suggestive procedures, including hypnosis and sodium pentothal (truth serum), the use of multiple psychotropic drugs, and an active search for "alters" and stories of abuse as contributing to the creation of false memories and a false disorder. Shows like *United States of Tara* further encourage disbelief by depicting a flamboyant and uncommon presentation of a woman who regularly engages in disturbing and unlikely behaviors in front of her children and others; all of this in spite of (or, perhaps, even because of) the show's employing Richard Kluft, who is a renowned expert in DID, as a consultant (Maron, 2009).

The *DSM*'s sole focus on alter personalities and the popular media portrayals give the impression that dissociated parts of the self regularly appear as separate people or that therapists consider these parts as different entities (Dell, 2006; Gleaves, 1996; Kluft, 1987). In fact, it is said to be extremely rare for an individual to present with overt behaviors of appearing as different people (Dell, 2009; Foote, 1999; Gleaves, 1996; Howell, 2011; Kluft, 2009; Spiegel et al., 2011), even though the subjective experience may be that they are different people or have different people living inside of them (International Society for the Study of Trauma and Dissociation, 2011; Tutkun, Yargic, & Sar, 1996).

Central to the construct of DID is a subjective, rather than overt, sense of separate entities, human or other, living inside one's body, experiences of something or someone possessing or controlling one's thoughts or actions, depersonalization, derealization, and amnesia for past and, possibly, present events that are not merely forgotten. Rather than considering dissociated parts of one's personality as truly separate entities, they may instead be conceptualized as metaphorical explanations of anomalous experiences that are attributed to internal, but depersonalized, parts of one's self (Merckelbach, Devilly, & Rassin, 2002). Although many dissociative disorder clinicians and researchers do not adopt this view, according to Putnam (1992), "reputable clinicians do not believe that the alter personalities represent distinct people" (p. 418).

Many within the trauma and dissociative disorder fields consider DID to lie on a continuum with PTSD and normality, though still existing as a separate disorder and still within the larger biomedical model. The structural theory of dissociation, which has become quite popular in this specialty field, proposes a continuum of a fractured psyche due to trauma (van der Hart, Nijenhuis, & Steele, 2006). The theory is based on Myers' (1940) observations of World War I soldiers who exhibited a split between what structural theorists (van der Hart, van Dijke, van Son, & Steele, 2001) call an emotional personality (EP) and an apparently normal personality (ANP). The EP is theorized to be stuck in the traumatic experiences, and the ANP is theorized to be characterized by amnesia, detachment, and numbing. Myers noted that there may be switching between these states wherein the EP intrudes upon the normal personality, only for the ANP to return with lack of memory for trauma-related distress or recall of the distress as dream-like or unreal. These traumatically divided parts of the personality have also been described in Holocaust survivors who continue to experience major distress even into their elderly years (Auerbach, Mirvis, Stern, & Schwartz, 2009). In particular, Auerbach et al. (2009) found that these survivors were characterized by an excessive reliance on the ANP, resulting in an emotionally absent lifestyle that lacked intimacy or significant attachment. Such a lifestyle may be adaptive by keeping the EP out of awareness, thereby allowing the person to function in daily life. This supports the idea that structural dissociation is a split between the system of defense and that which involves functioning and surviving in the present (Nijenhuis, van der Hart, & Steele, 2010).

The structurally dissociated parts of the personality are not considered to be truly separate entities, but are metaphoric constructs that describe these changes in the level of consciousness and awareness (van der Hart et al., 2001). The EP is most associated with traumatic re-experiencing, somatic sensations, traumatic memories, dissociated personality states, and psychotic experiences (Nijenhuis & van der Hart, 1999). The ANP is characterized by avoidance; episodes of amnesia; loss of sensory, perceptual, or motor functioning; depersonalization; and emotional numbness (Nijenhuis, Spinhoven, van Dyck, van der Hart, & Vanderlinden, 1996). These are also conceptualized as positive (intrusive) and negative (functional loss) symptoms of hyperarousal and inhibition (van der Hart et al., 2001).

This psychic division of an EP and ANP is considered to be primary structural dissociation that is associated with a single traumatic event and PTSD (van der Hart et al., 2006). In this model, the EP does not have a high level of autonomy and the ANP would mostly present as detached and numb (Steele, van der Hart, & Nijenhuis, 2005). However, as the traumatization becomes more severe and prolonged, and denial of the trauma increases, further divisions occur. Secondary structural dissociation is defined by a division of the EP and is associated with complex-PTSD (e.g., Herman, 2006), BPD, and dissociative disorders not otherwise specified. It is common for there to be a child-like EP fixated in trauma and another EP that may have observed the trauma from a detached position.

At the far end of this spectrum is what these theorists call tertiary structural dissociation, which is when the ANP is divided into two or more parts and multiple EPs exist, as is thought to be evident in DID. Each of these parts of the personality is purported to engage in distinct defenses, such as projection, denial, and splitting; however, they rename these defenses "mental coping strategies" in keeping with cognitive-behavioral ideology (Steele et al., 2005). Additionally, these parts are often in conflict and are extremely polarized. Persistence of these divisions is thought to act as different methods of phobic avoidance of traumatic memories (van der Hart et al., 2006).

We All Have Multiple Personalities

Psychodynamic Theory

> In accordance with my theme about recognizing that a person like me has many parts and that what is consciously expressed at any given time is far from the whole story, I wanted to address the issue of a client who discloses trauma, and then retracts it. I want therapists to realize how complicated the dynamics are regarding disclosure of trauma and abuse, specifically of a magnitude that would lead to severe dissociation. P13

In contrast to the structural DID theorists, it appears as though it is not trauma that causes a person to experience multiple selves, but rather all humans are multiple; it is more a degree of a subjective sense of fragmentation and depersonalization that distinguishes the trauma survivor. According to some more relationally focused psychoanalysts, for instance, there is no one self, but rather self-states that are consistent and fluid on a continuum of normalcy (Davies, 1996). Dissociation is seen as a central defense to overwhelming experience and exists within the relational process with others (Davies, 1996; Howell, 2005). The organization of the normal self, according to this theory, is not thought to be unitary, but rather a collection of different self-states that interact internally and interpersonally (Bradfield, 2011; Howell, 2011; Stern, 2003).

This is based on Harry Stack Sullivan's idea of the multiple self as universal and the self as existing only in an interpersonal context (Sullivan, 1954), which appears to be rooted in the writings of Janet (Davies, 1996). Sullivan (1954) believed that the self exists in relation to others, and therefore the multiplicity of the self exists in multiple relationships that elicit and require different self-states. When dissociation exists, parts of the self become disconnected from human contact and relatedness, preventing dialogue or conflict to exist within the whole self (Bradfield, 2011; Bromberg, 1998). Emotions, memories, and experience become separated to the point that they exist side by side, without awareness of a cohesive self, creating self-states that are distinct and omitted from auto-biographical memory (Bromberg, 2003). Everyone experiences this; think of the person who says "I'm never angry" and denies those moments where he or she inevitably is just that. The extent to which one experiences this, however, exists along a continuum of severity.

The organization of a traumatized individual's internal world mimics the dissociated experiences that the individual may be consciously unaware of (Stern, 1996). Each of these personified, dissociated, self-states develops around the relationship with self-states of particular significant people in the child's life (Stern, 2004), and have different representations of parental and familial objects and an organization of the ego that is specific to the age at which the trauma occurred (Davies, 1996). In other words, parts of the self become stuck in seeing the world and the people in it through the lens of these significant periods in the child's life. These disowned experiences and parts of the self become manifest through interactions wherein these early experiences are enacted both within the therapeutic relationship and in everyday life (Bromberg, 1995; Davies & Frawley, 1991).

An enactment is said to be the disavowal of aspects of the self and of internal conflict that is experienced, instead, by a vulnerable other who takes on these aspects (Stern, 2003). The experience of the therapist in relation to the client, or countertransference, can be an opportunity to discover and explore some of these unformulated and dissociated experiences and enactments (Davies & Frawley, 1991; Stern, 2004). At any given point, the therapist is likely to find his or her self in the role of perpetrator, rescuer, or victim, and ongoing themes of denial and identification will become manifest throughout the therapy process (Davies, 1996; Howell, 2011). This is a standard focus of relational therapy regardless of diagnosis, level of dissociation, or overt "symptoms".

It is thought by some interpersonal and relational therapists that the clinician's own multiplicity is what allows for observation of the countertransference and the awareness of the core self simultaneously (Stern, 2004). Multiplicity on the more typical end of the continuum is commonly evident in the experience of internal conflict, or of feeling different ways about the same thing. If this internal conflict is not experienced, but rather subjectively depersonalized and considered to be "not-me", the parts are said to be dissociated from one another. A major goal of therapy is to develop awareness of and tolerance for this internal conflict, thereby disbanding the need for enactments (Bromberg, 1998).

Internal Family Systems

> So what IFS does, it is a way of thinking and conducting therapy where you just assume that everybody exists in parts. We all have a social face we'll put in in one situation and we have parts like an inner child, kind of everyone has, everyone has that kind of stuff … there's conflict but it's like, ya know, a loving family. Whereas I guess the internal family is seen very much like an external dysfunctional family in a person who isn't functioning well. P13

Similar to the relational psychodynamic perspective, the Internal Family Systems (IFS) approach also considers multiplicity to be universal and lying on a continuum of severity and functionality. The IFS concept is non-pathologizing and strength-based, focusing on empowerment and understanding the contexts in which individual problems developed (Miller, Cardona, & Hardin, 2007). It originated from Schwartz's (1995) observations as a family systems clinician. He noticed that each of his clients exhibited disowned parts of themselves, whether it be their "angry parts", "loving parts", and so on, and he thought that family systems' techniques could be applicable in working with one's own internal family. Schwartz theorized that parts of the self form a complex system that mimic those in one's family, akin to the object relations theorists. Internal conflict and polarizations, or contrasting extreme beliefs or positions, that exist within everyone may be intensified by extreme conditions like trauma, chaos, denial, and abuse.

Three specific parts are described as existing in all people: (1) "managers" that are associated with functional living and safety, and tend to ignore problems; (2) "exiles" that are characterized by disowned experience and kept in isolation; and (3) "firefighters" that become active when exiles are triggered. In the traumatized individual, exiles hold the traumatic memories, and the associated extreme emotions and sensations, while firefighters may engage in impulsive and destructive behaviors to prevent the awareness of these repudiated events. In addition to these parts, everyone also is thought to have a core Self that innately has leadership qualities, including empathy, rational perspective, and acceptance. The parts are organized to protect this core Self (Pais, 2009).

In the case of more severe emotional distress, or experiences that might get labeled mentally ill, these parts become polarized, isolated, and protective in a disorganized fashion (Schwartz, 1995). Each part is thought to be fighting for control and attempts to deal with problems from its own narrow perspective. As in standard family systems theory, each member of the group is considered valuable and acting in a manner that is conducive to the context in which they live. All members are impacted by each other, and the entire system is impacted by one individual. Changing behavior in any one member will result in behavior changes in others due to this converging process of interacting parts. In this sense, extreme and harmful behaviors may be viewed as adaptive and protective actions conducted when the Self's abilities are not trusted to be in charge (Schwartz, 1995).

Neurology and Evolutionary Science

> I don't know how to explain it. It's like compartmentalizing in the brain I guess. P2

Findings from within the fields of neurology and evolutionary psychology also converge on the supposition that there is no one universal self, but rather that multiplicity is universal. What may separate those who get diagnosed from everyone else, beyond subjective distress, is not so much the multiplicity of self-states, but rather the phenomenon of hypnotic states in which the person is no longer in this world, is controllable and naïve, abruptly shifts between self-states with a lack of awareness or memory, and drifts in dream-like awareness.

Robert Kurzban is an evolutionary psychologist at the University of Pennsylvania whose work focuses on how cognition has adapted to function in a complex social world. In his book *Why Everyone Else is a Hypocrite* (Kurzban, 2010), he provides robust research and evidence to support his argument that "the human mind—and your mind—is modular, that it consists of a large number of specialized parts ... [that] can simultaneously hold different, mutually contradictory views, and there is nothing particularly odd or surprising about this" (p. 21). He describes how the mind actively keeps information compartmentalized and how some "modules" may not have access to such information even while others do. He states that "the large number of parts of the mind can be thought of as, in some sense, being different 'selves', designed to accomplish some task" (p. 9). This modularity is what helps explain such phenomena as self-deception and destruction, hypocrisy, and strategic ignorance, with scientists (and mental health professionals) particularly benefitting from splitting of the mind.

Neuroscience appears to support this theory of modularity of the mind as well. It appears that, at least within the brain, everyone has multiple personalities (Gazzaniga, 1988). Neurological research also supports the idea that the multiplicity of brain systems is what allows for moral reasoning and self-evaluative actions that may lead to alterations in behavior (Hitlin, 2008). In other words, multiplicity is what allows humans to function at the complex level they do.

While the concept of multiplicity is universal and exists on a continuum of severity of depersonalization ("not-me") experiences, individuals who might be diagnosed with DID are those who also experience a great deal of distressing phenomena in other dimensions. For instance, experiences more characteristic of and more commonly experienced by individuals with severe dissociation are: episodes of unexplainable physical ailments or even seizures, feeling like one is watching their life from outside his or her self, having "not-me" experiences, hearing voices, seeing things others cannot, trance states, identity confusion, experiences within the paranormal, and Schneiderian first-rank symptoms (Dell, 2006; Fink & Golinkoff, 1990; Howell, 2011; Kluft, 2009; Ross, 2011; Ross et al., 1990; Ross & Ness, 2010; Spiegel et al., 2011). Additionally, there is robust evidence demonstrating the link between dissociation and psychosis, generally (e.g., Pearce et al., 2017).

CAN PSYCHOSIS HEAL?

There's a big difference when you use certain terminology, and breakdown ... really needs to be changed ... [because] ... You're actually breaking through from an old pattern. P10

As discussed in Chap. 2, schizophrenia was long thought to be a condition of extreme ego-splitting and "not-me" experiences, which now appear to mostly fall under the category of DID. Yet, schizophrenia exists as a category describing a supposed genetic brain disease, while DID is often dismissed as unreal or the result of attention-seeking behaviors. Amazingly, theorists from all specialty areas of mental health keep inventing new terms to describe and separate "psychoses" that are dissociative or trauma-based while adhering to the faith-based ideology that such a thing as schizophrenia exists (e.g., Read, 1997). This allows the field to explain traumatic responses, such as voices, through a lens of dissociation, while never questioning the biological paradigm of 'schizophrenia' or defining what it even is (e.g., Moskowitz, 2011).

Interestingly, the structural theory of dissociation, despite its placement within a larger biomedical framework, provides a theoretical understanding as to how the structurally dissociated psyche and its associated intrusive thoughts, feelings, will, and behaviors that are depersonalized and compartmentalized may lend to the rise of so-called positive psychotic symptoms (e.g., Read, van Os, Morrison, & Ross, 2005). In fact, it is relatively common for severe psychotic phenomena to occur in individuals diagnosed with chronic PTSD (Hamner et al., 2000), and this may be related to reports of a greater number of traumatic experiences, more severe childhood trauma, and sexual abuse (e.g., Amsel, Hunter, Kim, Fodor, & Markowitz, 2012). At the same time, others purport that dissociation, itself, somehow "protects" people from a more pervasive psychosis because at any given moment one might "switch" into an altered state that is governed by completely different neuronal, cognitive, and affective pathways (Scharfetter, 2008). The idea is that severe dissociation may allow the person to appear "normal" during times of extreme detachment from experience, even when the internal process is, at times, identical to one deemed "psychotic".

Yet, individuals who are considered to have experienced acute psychosis maintain insight into their experience until well into the breakdown process (Birchwood, Mason, MacMillan, & Healy, 1993), and a "fear of going crazy" is the most common prodromal symptom (Hirsch & Jolley, 1989). It is also common for voice-hearers to attribute their voices to dissociated parts of the self as they begin to make meaning of these experiences and confront their traumatic histories (Romme, Escher, Dillon, Corstens, & Morris, 2009). Cooke and Kinderman (2017) argue that no matter how strange a person's behaviors or belief system may be, it almost always can be understood psychologically. Additionally, it has been discussed in countless psychoanalytic texts that even those in the most extreme states of psychosis still have "islands of clarity" wherein they can maintain a foot in both their world and that of consensual reality (Karon, 2000).

Schizophrenia may actually be understood through a conceptual framework based on dissociation, and this is supported by neuroimaging studies (Bob & Mashour, 2011). In concordance with this, some first-person accounts of recovery from psychosis (Boevink & Corstens, 2012; Dillon, 2012) and therapists working psychosocially with psychosis (Bacon & Kennedy, 2015) assert that psychosis and dissociation are different concepts but not separate; rather, both are understandable, interrelated, and meaningful parallel human reactions to severe childhood trauma. Pope and Kwapil (2000) found that dissociative experiences are positively correlated with psychosis proneness, generally, which further suggests the non-distinct nature of these two categories (Freeman & Garety, 2003), no matter how poorly defined either are.

In other words, far from being a pathological disease process, entering altered states and experiencing sensations without external stimuli may be the body's very natural attempt to heal and process experiences that are otherwise too overwhelming to contain. Allen, Coyne, and Console (1997) found that dissociative detachment from one's actions, self, and environment was related to "thought disorder", so-called delusional thinking, severe confusion, disorganization, and disorientation, rendering individuals vulnerable to psychosis. Startup (1999) has shown that the general population exhibits phenomena that are postulated as definitive of both psychotic and dissociative in continuously variable and non-pathological forms.

Psychosis, like all mental phenomena, is demonstrated to exist on a continuum in the general population (Collip et al., 2013; Shevlin, Boyda, Houston, & Murphy, 2015). In fact, it has been found that a history of hearing voices and delusional thinking is common in people who have never had any psychiatric history or dysfunction at all (McGrath et al., 2015), and that such experiences are related to emotional reactivity and stress (Collip et al., 2013). Approximately 3% to 20% of the general public experiences auditory hallucinations (Beavan, Read, & Cartwright, 2011). Voices have also been found to lie on a continuum of experience from normal to severe, largely based on the level of distress associated with the experience (Honig et al., 1998) and the meaning one attributes to these experiences (Peters et al., 2017). Furthermore, voices may also be considered as situated along a continuum with dissociated parts of the self, depending on the level of autonomy associated with specific voices and their ability to subjectively take executive control (Peterson, 1995). Voices, like dissociated parts, are thought to represent emotional conflicts that have been disowned (Corstens & Longden, 2013), and, in fact, are predicted by levels of dissociation (Moskowitz & Corstens, 2007; Varese, Udachina, Myin-Germeys, Oorschot, & Bentall, 2011).

If so-called psychotic phenomena were perceived as responses to adversity and stress, then it is not a leap to consider the potential healing potential of the psychotic experience. Although controversial, discussion of the transformative power of psychosis has been ongoing since at least the time of Carl Jung (1939–1961). Jung, like many other analysts of the early twentieth century, believed that schizophrenia (or dementia praecox as it was then known) was a condition resulting from an extreme dissociation of the multiple selves and a process of entering dream-like states while awake. These extreme states offered an opportunity to interpret the unconscious communications and conflicts symbolized through imagery and archetypes evident in the dream and characters depicted by the multiple selves. Put more simply, Jung believed the psychotic process offers an opportunity for understanding and transformation. More recent qualitative studies with individuals who identify as having recovered from psychosis also suggest that psychosis is part of a transformational process that can lead to an increased sense of mindfulness, spirituality, and empowerment (e.g., Hagen & Nixon, 2010; Nixon, Hagen, & Peters, 2010).

Ironically, while the mental health field continues to promote a biomedical understanding of "schizophrenia", they are simultaneously endorsing increased focus on using psychedelics to "treat" people diagnosed with depression, PTSD, and more. In other words, they are finding increasing evidence that psychotic experience can be medicinal. Of course, taking a substance in a supervised and controlled setting for a limited time period is different than prolonged distress without support or direction. Yet, the idea that naturally occurring psychotic experiences are somehow sick while drug-induced psychosis (clarification: legal, prescribed drug-induced psychosis supervised by a professional expert) is somehow medicine is not a given fact. The evidence appears to indicate quite the opposite.

Since the beginning of time, humans have been using substances to heal, numb pain, and enhance spiritual experience and meaning in life. Many shamanic and spiritual traditions, such as Shamanism, Hinduism, and Rastafarianism, have long used hallucinogens to expand consciousness, find empowerment, escape oppression, connect with others, and promote religious connection and vision. The modern religion of psychiatry is now also discovering the healing potential of these substances.

Far from being a benign experience, participants of studies on psychedelics report periods of extensive fear and anxiety (MacLean, Johnson, & Griffiths, 2011), and confusion and "thought disorder" (Carhart-Harris et al., 2017). Rather than these experiences being detrimental, individuals who reported this more severe distress were actually those who demonstrated the greatest transformation and healing. Further, mystical experiences and the meaning-making of the psychedelic experience are said to be critical elements determining a positive experience of the psychotic process in these studies (e.g., Tupper, Wood, Yensen, & Johnson, 2015).

Psychedelic drugs have been suggested to offer potential not only to heal from anxiety, depression, suicidality, and trauma (Carhart-Harris et al., 2017; Oehen, Traber, Widmer, & Schnyder, 2012; Shroder, 2014), they also are thought to offer protection from emotional difficulties (Palhano-Fontes et al., 2017) and prevention of suicide (Hendricks,

Thorne, Clark, Coombs, & Johnson, 2015). Use of psychedelics has been shown to result in lasting personality change (MacLean et al., 2011) and decreased substance use (Thomas, Lucas, Capler, Tupper, & Martin, 2013). Of course, the use of psychedelic drugs is only promoted by professionals when prescribed by professionals; recreational abuse continues to be considered bad (Palhano-Fontes et al., 2017) as does a naturally occurring psychedelic experience (i.e., "psychosis").

EVERYONE IS DELUSIONAL

I would say that arguing with a paranoid about their delusions is probably futile. It's a waste of your energy because you're not going to change their [minds] ... it would be better if you just let them talk to you about the delusion and not necessarily try to combat it with what you see as the facts. Or what may be the facts that this person doesn't see. P2

It is so much easier to believe that I am crazy and that I had a perfect childhood with parents who loved me and simply got worn out from dealing with a mentally sick daughter like me, than it is to come to terms with the fact that the definition of love does not make allowances for the things that happened, and that my perfect childhood is not in accordance with my memories, somatic and otherwise. P13

Semantics and cultural norms have a lot to do with how a belief system is determined to be ignorant, atypical, metaphysical, spiritual, religious, superstitious, illusory, or delusional. There is no objective truth that separates these various descriptions of beliefs that may not be in accord with consensus reality. In general, however, a delusion is considered to be a belief that is fixed despite contradictory evidence, qualified as either *bizarre* or *non-bizarre*. As with religions of yore, psychiatry tells society what is acceptable and not to believe, and if a person does not conform, they are frequently cast out (hospitalized) and condemned as a heretic (delusional). Even with this, up to 70% of the general population have belief systems that could be labeled delusional (Verdoux et al., 1998).

It is frequently suggested by dissociative specialists that, though overlapping in many regards, the true difference between DID and schizophrenia is the presence of "delusions". For instance, some (e.g., Laddis & Dell, 2012; Spiegel et al., 2011) propose that individuals who are diagnosed with a traumatic or dissociative disorder often tend to attribute their psychotic experiences to parts of the self, rather than reporting "bizarre" delusional explanations that have no psychological precedence or reality-based truth. They do this, of course, by utilizing questionnaires that are based on the premise that bizarre delusions are not dissociative and showing that, indeed, dissociation is not related to bizarre delusions (this is called tautological reasoning). In spite of this, some have actually found strong associations of so-called delusional thinking with dissociation (Spitzer, Haug, & Freyberger, 1997).

Similar to everything discussed thus far, delusional and paranoid thinking may also be considered as lying on a continuum with typical experiences, again with level of distress associated with the level of dysfunction (Cafferkey, Murphy, & Shevlin, 2014; Peters, Joseph, Day, & Garety, 2004). Cognitive distortions, biases, and errors exist within all individuals (including clinicians!) to a greater or lesser degree, and trauma, emotional neglect, and/or chronic stress may result in extreme and rigid cognitive errors or fantasies that could be considered "delusional" by one who does not understand (see Bentall, 2003). While it may seem apparent to the professional who is indoctrinated into seeing "disease" based on superficial "symptoms" that rationalization of internal experiences couched in terms of parts of the self versus, for example, radioactive waves from the television is clearly a different phenomenon, the process underlying these explanations may not be. In fact, the only difference may be the cultural acceptance of one explanation over another, the obviousness of its relationship to overt trauma, and the clinician's ability to understand (e.g., Morrison, Frame, & Larkin, 2003).

Even using the clinical, standard construct of delusion, it has been demonstrated that approximately 1% to 3% of the general public are considered to have delusions at a severity level indicative of psychosis, yet without requiring any treatment (Freeman, 2006). Freeman (2006) found that a further 5% to 6% of the non-clinical population experienced less severe delusions associated with social and emotional difficulties, and 10% to 15% of the population has regular delusional ideation. A separate study by Pechey and Halligan (2011) found that 39% of the general population experiences delusional beliefs, with 25% reporting "bizarre" delusions. It appears as though delusional (and hallucinatory) experiences are more common in college students than the general population (Lincoln & Keller, 2008). These delusional experiences are not so "bizarre", though, when considering that they tend to be associated with severity levels of anxiety and depression, even in the general population (Saha, Scott, Varghese, & McGrath, 2012).

Interestingly, perhaps, is a theory put forth by Hugh Jones (Jones, Delespaul, & van Os, 2003) that the modularity of the mind (multiplicity; Fodor, 1983) is what allows for delusions to exist in the first place. He proposes that "normal" beliefs must be accessible to all modules in order to function, but that delusions are those that are encapsulated in particular modules. If one were to consider the adaptive nature of this process, as Laing did 60 years ago, it can be seen that due to various circumstances one self-part may hold a particular belief in order to protect the greater whole self. So, for instance, one may refuse to acknowledge or consider evidence contradictory to his or her beliefs if it threatens a caregiver, threatens flooding of emotion, threatens unbearable ambiguity or uncertainty, threatens a worldview, or threatens one's career.

Where is the line between an *irrational belief* (common to all humans) and a *delusion* (an alleged sign of illness)? Is the belief that a man died, arose from the dead three days later, and absolved the world of its sins a delusion or just a religious belief? Is the belief that a child is supposed to sit still and quiet without physical activity for hours on end attending to boring tasks a delusion or just an ideological societal belief? It may be stated, especially by trauma specialists, that delusions are bizarre and completely implausible (e.g., Laddis & Dell, 2012). Yet, who has the authority to decide what is irrational versus bizarre, religious versus insane, trauma-based versus brain disease? Modern society dictates that it is the psychiatrist; previous decades have given such privileges to priests, shamans, kings, emperors, and rabbis. Is this objective science?

REFERENCES

Allen, J., Coyne, L., & Console, D. A. (1997). Dissociative detachment relates to psychotic symptoms and personality decompensation. *Comprehensive Psychiatry, 38*, 327–334.

Amsel, L. V., Hunter, N., Kim, S., Fodor, K. E., & Markowitz, J. C. (2012). Does a study focused on trauma encourage patients with psychotic symptoms to seek treatment? *Psychiatric Services, 63*(4), 386–389.

Auerbach, C. F., Mirvis, S., Stern, S., & Schwartz, J. (2009). Structural dissociation and its resolution among Holocaust survivors: A qualitative research study. *Journal of Trauma & Dissociation, 10*(4), 385–404.

Bacon, T., & Kennedy, A. (2015). Clinical perspectives on the relationship between psychosis and dissociation: Utility of structural dissociation and implications for practice. *Psychosis, 7*(1), 81–91.

Beavan, V., Read, J., & Cartwright, C. (2011). The prevalence of voice-hearers in the general population: A literature review. *Journal of Mental Health, 20*(3), 281–292. https://doi.org/10.3109/09638237.2011.562262

Bentall, R. P. (2003). *Madness explained: Psychosis and human nature*. London: Penguin.

Birchwood, M., Mason, R., MacMillan, F., & Healy, J. (1993). Depression, demoralization and control of psychotic illness: A comparison of depressed and nondepressed patients with a chronic psychosis. *Psychological Medicine, 23*, 387–395.

Bob, P., & Mashour, G. A. (2011). Schizophrenia, dissociation, and consciousness. *Consciousness and Cognition, 20*(4), 1042–1049.

Boevink, W., & Corstens, D. (2012). My body remembers; I refused: Childhood trauma, dissociation and psychosis. In J. Geekie, D. Randal, D. Lampshire, & J. Read (Eds.), *Experiencing psychosis* (pp. 119–126). New York: Routledge.

Bradfield, B. (2011). Dissociation and restoration in trauma survivors and their children. *Psychoanalytic Psychotherapy in South Africa, 19*(2), 66–102.

Bromberg, P. M. (1995). Resistance, object usage, and human relatedness. *Contemporary Psychoanalysis, 31*(2), 173–191.

Bromberg, P. M. (1998). *Standing in the spaces: Essays on clinical process, trauma, and dissociation*. Hillsdale, NJ: The Analytic Press.

Bromberg, P. M. (2003). One need not be a house to be haunted: On enactment, dissociation, and the dread of "not-me" – A case study. *Psychoanalytic Dialogues, 13*, 689–709.

Cafferkey, K., Murphy, J., & Shevlin, M. (2014). Jumping to conclusions: The association between delusional ideation and reasoning biases in a healthy student population. *Psychosis, 6*(3), 206–214. https://doi.org/10.1080/175224 39.2013.850734

Carhart-Harris, R. L., Roseman, L., Bolstridge, M., Demetriou, L., Pannekoek, J. N., Wall, M. B., ... Nutt, D. J. (2017). Psilocybin for treatment-resistant depression: fMRI-measured brain mechanisms. *Scientific Reports, 7*(1), 13187. https://doi.org/10.1038/s41598-017-13282-7

Collip, D., Wigman, J. T., Myin-Germeys, I., Jacobs, N., Derom, C., Thiery, E., ... van Os, J. (2013). From epidemiology to daily life: Linking daily life stress reactivity to persistence of psychotic experiences in a longitudinal general population study. *PLoS ONE, 8*(4), e62688. https://doi.org/10.1371/journal.pone.0062688

Cooke, A., & Kinderman, P. (2017). "But what about real mental illnesses?" Alternatives to the disease model approach to "schizophrenia". *Journal of Humanistic Psychology, 58*(1), 47–71. https://doi.org/10.1177/0022167817745621

Corstens, D., & Longden, E. (2013). The origins of voices: Links between life history and voice hearing in a survey of 100 cases. *Psychosis, 5*(3), 270–285. https://doi.org/10.1080/17522439.2013.816337

Crosby, A. E., Han, B., Ortega, L. A. G., Parks, S. E., & Gfroerer, J. (2011). Suicidal thoughts and behaviors among adults aged ≥18 years – United States, 2008–2009. *Morbidity and Mortality Weekly Report (MMWR)*. Retrieved from https://www.cdc.gov/mmwr/preview/mmwrhtml/ss6013a1.htm

Davies, J. M. (1996). Dissociation, repression and reality testing in the counter-transference: The controversey over memory and false memory in the psycho-analytic treatment of adult survivors of childhood sexual abuse. *Psychoanalytic Dialogues, 6*(2), 189–218.

Davies, J. M., & Frawley, M. G. (1991). Dissociative processes and transference-countertransference paradigms in the psychoanalytically oriented treatment of adult survivors of childhood sexual abuse. *Psychoanalytic Dialogues, 2*, 5–36.

Dell, P. F. (2006). A new model of dissociative identity disorder. *Psychiatric Clinics of North America, 29*(1), 1–26 vii.

Dell, P. F. (2009). The phenomena of pathological dissociation. In P. F. Dell & J. A. O'Neil (Eds.), *Dissociation and the dissociative disorders: DSM-V and beyond* (pp. 228–238). New York: Routledge.

Dillon, J. (2012). Recovery from 'psychosis'. In J. Geekie, P. Randal, D. Lampshire, & J. Read (Eds.), *Experiencing psychosis*. New York, NY: Routledge.

Fink, D., & Golinkoff, M. (1990). MPD, borderline personality disorder and schizophrenia: A comparative study of clinical features. *Dissociation, 3*, 127–134.

Fodor, J. A. (1983). *Modularity of mind*. Cambridge, MA: MIT Press.

Foote, B. (1999). Dissociative identity disorder and pseudo-hysteria. *American Journal of Psychotherapy, 53*(3), 320–343.

Freeman, D. (2006). Delusions in the nonclinical population. *Current Psychiatry Reports, 8*(3), 191–204.

Freeman, D., & Garety, P. A. (2003). Connecting neurosis and psychosis: The direct influence of emotion on delusions and hallucinations. *Behavior Research and Therapy, 41*(8), 923–947.

Gazzaniga, M. S. (1988). *The Social Brain: Discovering the Networks of the Mind*. New York: Basic Books.

Gleaves, D. H. (1996). The sociocognitive model of dissociative identity disorder: A reexamination of the evidence. *Psychological Bulletin, 120*(1), 42–59.

Hagen, B., & Nixon, G. (2010). Psychosis as a potentially transformative experience: Implications for psychologists and counsellors. *Procedia Social and Behavioral Sciences, 5*, 722–726.

Hamner, M. B., Frueh, B. C., Ulmer, H. G., Huber, M. G., Twomey, T. J., Tyson, C., & Arana, G. W. (2000). Psychotic features in chronic posttraumatic stress disorder and schizophrenia: Comparative severity. *Journal of Nervous and Mental Disease, 188*, 217–221.

Hendricks, P. S., Thorne, C. B., Clark, C. B., Coombs, D. W., & Johnson, M. W. (2015). Classic psychedelic use is associated with reduced psychological distress and suicidality in the United States adult population. *Journal of Psychopharmacology, 29*(3), 280–288.

Herman, J. (2006). Complex PTSD: A syndrome in survivors of prolonged and repeated trauma. *Journal of Traumatic Stress, 5,* 377–391.

Hirsch, S. R., & Jolley, A. G. (1989). The dysphoric syndrome in schizophrenia and its implications for relapse. *British Journal of Psychiatry, 156,* 46–50.

Hitlin, S. (2008). Evolution, society, and conscience: Social influences on morality. In *Moral selves, evil selves: The social psychology of conscience* (pp. 53–74). New York: Palgrave Macmillan.

Honig, A., Romme, M., Ensink, B., Escher, S., Pennings, M., & Devries, M. (1998). Auditory hallucinations: A comparison between patients and nonpatients. *Journal of Nervous and Mental Disease, 186*(10), 646–651.

Howell, E. (2005). *The dissociative mind.* London: Routledge.

Howell, E. (2011). *Understanding and treating dissociative identity disorder: A relational approach.* New York, NY: Taylor and Francis Group, LLC.

Hunter, N. (2015). Clinical trainees' personal history of suicidality and the effects on attitudes towards suicidal patients. *The New School Psychology Bulletin, 13*(1), 38–46.

International Society for the Study of Trauma and Dissociation. (2011). Guidelines for treating dissociative identity disorder in adults, third revision. [Practice Guideline]. *Journal of Trauma & Dissociation, 12*(2), 115–187.

Jones, H., Delespaul, P., & van Os, J. (2003). Jaspers was right after all – Delusions are distinct from normal beliefs. *The British Journal of Psychiatry, 183*(4), 285–286.

Jung, C. G. (Ed.). (1939/1961). *On the psychogenesis of schizophrenia* (Vol. 3). New York: Routledge.

Karon, B. P. (2000). *Effective psychoanalytic therapy of schizophrenia and other severe disorders.* Washington, DC: American Psychological Association.

Kluft, R. P. (1987). First rank symptoms as diagnostic indicators of multiple personality disorder. *American Journal of Psychiatry, 144,* 293–298.

Kluft, R. P. (2009). A clinician's understanding of dissociation: Fragments of an acquaintance. In P. F. Dell & J. A. O'Neil (Eds.), *Dissociation and the dissociative disorders: DSM-V and beyond.* New York: Routledge.

Kurzban, R. (2010). *Why everyone (else) is a hypocrite.* Princeton, NJ: Princeton University Press.

Laddis, A., & Dell, P. F. (2012). Dissociation and psychosis in dissociative identity disorder and schizophrenia. *Journal of Trauma & Dissociation, 13*(4), 397–413.

Lincoln, T. M., & Keller, E. (2008). Delusions and hallucinations in students compared to the general population. *Psychology and Psychotherapy: Theory, Research and Practice, 81*(3), 231–235.

Liotti, G., & Gumley, A. (2008). An attachment perspective on schizophrenia: The role of disorganized attachment, dissociation and mentalization. In A. Moskowitz,

I. Schafer, & M. J. Dorahy (Eds.), *Psychosis, trauma and dissociation: Emerging perspectives on severe psychopathology* (pp. 117–133). West Sussex: John Wiley & Sons, Ltd.

MacLean, K. A., Johnson, M. W., & Griffiths, R. R. (2011). Mystical experiences occasioned by the hallucinogen psilocybin lead to increases in the personality domain of openness. *Journal of Psychopharmacology, 25*(11), 1453–1461.

Maron, D. F. (2009). TV's split personality. *Newsweek*. Retrieved from www.thedailybeast.com/newsweek

McGrath, J. J., Saha, S., Al-Hamzawi, A., Alonso, J., Bromet, E. J., Bruffaerts, R., … Kessler, R. C. (2015). Psychotic experiences in the general population: A cross-national analysis based on 31261 respondents from 18 countries. *JAMA Psychiatry.* https://doi.org/10.1001/jamapsychiatry.2015.0575

Merckelbach, H., Devilly, G. J., & Rassin, E. (2002). Alters in dissociative identity disorder metaphors or genuine entities? *Clinical Psychology Review, 22*(4), 481–498.

Miller, B. J., Cardona, J. R. P., & Hardin, M. (2007). The use of narrative therapy and internal family systems with survivors of childhood sexual abuse. *Journal of Feminist Family Therapy, 18*(4), 1–27.

Morrison, A. P., Frame, L., & Larkin, W. (2003). Relationships between trauma and psychosis: A review and integration. *British Journal of Clinical Psychology, 42*, 331–353.

Moskowitz, A. (2011). Schizophrenia, trauma, dissociation, and scientific revolutions. [Editorial]. *Journal of Trauma & Dissociation, 12*(4), 347–357.

Moskowitz, A., & Corstens, D. (2007). Auditory hallucinations: Psychotic symptom or dissociative experience? *Journal of Psychological Trauma, 6*, 35–63.

Myers, C. S. (1940). *Shell shock in France 1914–18.* Cambridge: Cambridge University Press.

Nathan, D. (2011). *Sybil exposed: The extraordinary story behind the famous multiple personality case.* New York: Free Press.

Nijenhuis, E. R., Spinhoven, P., van Dyck, R., van der Hart, O., & Vanderlinden, J. (1996). The development and psychometric characteristics of the Somatoform Dissociation Questionnaire (SDQ-20). *Journal of Nervous and Mental Disease, 184*, 688–694.

Nijenhuis, E. R., & van der Hart, O. (1999). Somatoform dissociative phenomena: A Janetian perspective. In J. Goodwin & R. Attias (Eds.), *Splintered reflections: Images of the body in trauma* (pp. 89–127). New York: Basic Books.

Nijenhuis, E. R., van der Hart, O., & Steele, K. (2010). Trauma-related structural dissociation of the personality. *Activitas Nervosa Superior, 52*, 1–23.

Nixon, G., Hagen, B., & Peters, T. (2010). Psychosis and transformation: A phenomenological inquiry. *International Journal of Mental Health and Addiction, 8*, 527–544.

Nock, M. K., Borges, G., Bromet, E. J., Alonso, J., Angermeyer, M., Beautrais, A., … Williams, D. R. (2008). Cross-national prevalence and risk factors for suicidal ideation, plans, and attempts. *The British Journal of Psychiatry: The Journal of Mental Science, 192,* 98–105. https://doi.org/10.1192/bjp.bp.107.040113

Oehen, P., Traber, R., Widmer, V., & Schnyder, U. (2012). A randomized, controlled pilot study of MDMA (±3,4-methylenedioxymethamphetamine)-assisted psychotherapy for treatment of resistant, chronic Post-Traumatic Stress Disorder (PTSD). *Journal of Psychopharmacology, 27*(1), 40–52. https://doi.org/10.1177/0269881112464827

Pais, S. (2009). A systematic approach to the treatment of dissociative identity disorder. *Journal of Family Psychotherapy, 20*(1), 72–88.

Palhano-Fontes, F., Barreto, D., Onias, H., Andrade, K. C., Novaes, M., Pessoa, J., … de Araujo, D. B. (2017). Rapid antidepressant effects of the psychedelic ayahuasca in treatment-resistant depression: A randomised placebo-controlled trial. *bioRxiv.* https://doi.org/10.1101/103531

Patel, V., Flisher, A. J., Hetrick, S., & McGorry, P. (2007). Mental health of young people: A global public-health challenge. *The Lancet, 369*(9569), 1302–1313 https://doi.org/10.1016/S0140-6736(07)60368-7

Pearce, J., Simpson, J., Berry, K., Bucci, S., Moskowitz, A., & Varese, F. (2017). Attachment and dissociation as mediators of the link between childhood trauma and psychotic experiences. *Clinical Psychology & Psychotherapy, 24*(6), 1304–1312.

Pechey, R., & Halligan, P. (2011). The prevalence of delusion-like beliefs relative to sociocultural beliefs in the general population. *Psychopathology, 44,* 106–115.

Peters, E., Joseph, S. A., Day, S., & Garety, P. A. (2004). Measuring delusional ideation: The 21-item Peters et al. Delusions Inventory (PDI). *Schizophrenia Bulletin, 30,* 1005–1022.

Peters, E., Ward, T., Jackson, M., Woodruff, P., Morgan, C., McGuire, P., & Garety, P. A. (2017). Clinical relevance of appraisals of persistent psychotic experiences in people with and without a need for care: An experimental study. *The Lancet Psychiatry, 4*(12), 927–936. https://doi.org/10.1016/s2215-0366(17)30409-1

Peterson, G. (1995). Auditory hallucinations and dissociative identity disorder [Letter to the Editor]. *American Journal of Psychiatry, 152*(9), 1403.

Pope, C. A., & Kwapil, T. R. (2000). Dissociative experiences in hypothetically psychosis-prone college students. *Journal of Nervous and Mental Disease, 188,* 530–536.

Putnam, F. W. (1992). Letter to the editor. *British Journal of Psychiatry, 161,* 417–418.

Read, J. (1997). Child abuse and psychosis: A literature review and implications for professionals. *Professional Psychology: Research and Practice, 28*(5), 448–456.

Read, J., van Os, J., Morrison, A. P., & Ross, C. A. (2005). Childhood trauma, psychosis, and schizophrenia: A literature review with theoretical and clinical implications. *Acta Psychiatrica Scandinavica, 112*, 330–350.

Rieber, R. W. (2006). *The bifurcation of the self: The history and theory of dissociation and its disorders.* New York: Springer.

Romme, M., Escher, S., Dillon, J., Corstens, D., & Morris, M. (Eds.). (2009). *Living with voices: 50 stories of recovery.* Herefordshire: PCCS Books Ltd.

Ross, C. A. (1990). Twelve cognitive errors about multiple personality disorder. *American Journal of Psychotherapy, 44,* 348–356.

Ross, C. A. (2007). *The trauma model: A solution to the problem of comorbidity in psychiatry.* Richardson, TX: Manitou Communications, Inc.

Ross, C. A. (2011). Possession experiences in dissociative identity disorder: A preliminary study. *Journal of Trauma & Dissociation, 12*(4), 393–400.

Ross, C. A., Miller, S. D., Reagor, P., Bjornson, L., Fraser, G. A., & Anderson, G. (1990). Schneiderian symptoms in multiple personality disorder and schizophrenia. *Comprehensive Psychiatry, 31*(2), 111–118.

Ross, C. A., & Ness, L. (2010). Symptom patterns in dissociative identity disorder patients and the general population. *Journal of Trauma & Dissociation, 11*(4), 458–468.

Saha, S., Scott, J., Varghese, D., & McGrath, J. J. (2012). Anxiety and depressive disorders are associated with delusional-like experiences: A replication study based on a National Survey of Mental Health and Wellbeing. *BMJ Open, 2*(3), e001001. https://doi.org/10.1136/bmjopen-2012-001001

Scharfetter, C. (2008). Ego-fragmentation in schizophrenia: A severe dissociation of self-experience. In A. Moskowitz, I. Schafer, & M. J. Dorahy (Eds.), *Psychosis, trauma and dissociation: Emerging perspectives on severe psychopathology* (pp. 51–64). West Sussex: John Wiley & Sons, Ltd.

Schwartz, R. C. (1995). *Internal family systems therapy.* New York: Guilford.

Shevlin, M., Boyda, D., Houston, J., & Murphy, J. (2015). Measurement of the psychosis continuum: Modelling the frequency and distress of subclinical psychotic experiences. *Psychosis, 7*(2), 108–118.

Shroder, T. (2014). *Acid test: LSD, ecstasy, and the power to heal.* New York: Penguin Group.

Spiegel, D., Loewenstein, R. J., Lewis-Fernandez, R., Sar, V., Simeon, D., Vermetten, E., ... Dell, P. F. (2011). Dissociative disorders in DSM-5. *Depression and Anxiety, 28*(9), 824–852.

Spitzer, C., Haug, H. J., & Freyberger, H. J. (1997). Dissociative symptoms in schizophrenic patients with positive and negative symptoms. *Psychopathology, 30,* 67–75.

Startup, M. (1999). Schizotypy, dissociative experiences and childhood abuse: Relationships among self-report measures. *British Journal of Clinical Psychology, 38,* 333–344.

Steele, K., van der Hart, O., & Nijenhuis, E. R. (2005). Phase-oriented treatment of structural dissociation in complex traumatization: Overcoming trauma-related phobias. *Journal of Trauma & Dissociation, 6*, 11–53.

Stern, D. B. (1996). Dissociation and constructivism: Commentary on papers by Davies and Harris. *Psychoanalytic Dialogues, 6*(2), 251–266.

Stern, D. B. (2003). The fusion of horizons: Dissociation, enactment, and understanding. *Psychoanalytic Dialogues, 13*, 843–873.

Stern, D. B. (2004). The eye sees itself: Dissociation, enactment, and the achievement of conflict. *Contemporary Psychoanalysis, 40*, 197–237.

Sullivan, H. S. (1954). *The interpersonal theory of psychiatry.* New York: Norton and Company, Inc.

Thomas, G., Lucas, P., Capler, N. R., Tupper, K. W., & Martin, G. N. (2013). Ayahuasca-assisted therapy for addiction: Results from a preliminary observational study in Canada. *Current Drug Abuse Reviews, 6*, 30–42.

Tupper, K. W., Wood, E., Yensen, R., & Johnson, M. W. (2015). Psychedelic medicine: A re-emerging therapeutic paradigm. *Canadian Medical Association Journal.* https://doi.org/10.1503/cmaj.141124

Tutkun, H., Yargic, L., & Sar, V. (1996). Dissociative identity disorder presenting as hysterical psychosis. *Dissociation, 9*, 241–249.

van der Hart, O., Nijenhuis, E. R., & Steele, K. (2006). *The haunted self: Structural dissociation and the treatment of chronic traumatization.* New York, NY: W. W. Norton.

van der Hart, O., van Dijke, A., van Son, M., & Steele, K. (2001). Somatoform dissociation in traumatized World War I combat soldiers. *Journal of Trauma & Dissociation, 1*(4), 33–66.

Varese, F., Udachina, A., Myin-Germeys, I., Oorschot, M., & Bentall, R. P. (2011). The relationship between dissociation and auditory verbal hallucinations in the flow of daily life of patients with psychosis. *Psychosis, 3*(1), 14–28.

Verdoux, H., Maurice-Tison, S., Gay, B., Van Os, J., Salamon, R., & Bourgeois, M. L. (1998). A survey of delusional ideation in primary-care patients. *Psychological Medicine, 28*(1), 127–134.

World Health Organization. (n.d.). Mental health: Data and statistics. Retrieved from http://www.euro.who.int/en/health-topics/noncommunicable-diseases/mental-health/data-and-statistics

CHAPTER 6

The Body and Mind in Context: The Role of Trauma and Adversity

I became very attached to this idea that all that had happened to me was a spiritual emergence, that I was a shaman-in-training, and that I had never been abused, that I'd had the perfect childhood, etcetera.... Coming to terms with the fact that my memories of my history and its present-day effects are not simply delusions has been one of the most heartbreaking things I had ever done. P13

Chronic stress, relative poverty, racism, oppression, social marginalization, child abuse, multiple types of trauma, and problems in attachment to caregivers contribute to a complex interplay of risk factors for suicidality, depression, altered states of consciousness, hearing or seeing things others do not, and fragmentation of one's sense of self. The role of trauma is frequently denied by many mental health professionals, society, and one's self alike, while individuals suffering from the after-effects, in turn, have great difficulty in obtaining the help and support they need to heal from what some refer to as *soul-wounds* (e.g., Duran, Firehammer, & Gonzalez, 2008). Somehow, it is controversial to suggest that what is being observed with "mental illness" generally is, in fact, a unique constellation of understandable and adaptive reactions to overwhelming and unbearable experiences. Rather, leaders in mental health would have us believe that we are helpless pawns of our genetic and biochemical will, reduced to neurons firing, as a car might be reduced to its engine.

Although there are many postulations regarding potential genetic and biological findings related to categories such as schizophrenia or bipolar

© The Author(s) 2018
N. Hunter, *Trauma and Madness in Mental Health Services*,
https://doi.org/10.1007/978-3-319-91752-8_6

disorder, the few findings reported thus far that have not been refuted are those that demonstrate minor differences across hundreds of genomic and neurological sites. Further, these findings are only significant in large populations (as opposed to the individual level) and cannot be differentiated from environmental effects of stress, trauma, and childhood adversity (e.g., Read, Fosse, Moskowitz, & Perry, 2014; Richardson, 2017).

Aside from the effects directly linked to psychotropic drug use, findings demonstrating altered brain patterns for individuals who are said to have experienced psychosis appear to only be found in those who also have specifically experienced child abuse (Teicher & Samson, 2016). These same brain patterns are also found in individuals and children who have experienced abuse but who have not had any diagnosable psychiatric difficulties (Read et al., 2014). And, even with these biological differences found for some groups of people, lifestyle changes, such as a healthy diet, forming and maintaining supportive relationships, psychotherapy, yoga, meditation, and exercise, have all been demonstrated to have the ability to alter brain structures and even genetic expression in a healthier direction.

While this may not be entirely surprising for experiences such as depression, anxiety, and suicidality, it is often taken for granted that "serious mental illness" is something different. This myth (see Chap. 4) is perpetuated by trauma and dissociative disorder specialists as well, thereby allowing, of course, the status quo to be maintained and the overarching ideological paradigm (see Chap. 3) to go unchallenged in the face of overwhelming evidence demonstrating the effects of trauma and adversity in all its varied forms. Yet, a myth it is, and the evidence continues to accumulate, making it nearly irrefutable that most often what is being perceived by the most "serious" of "serious mental illnesses" are actually responses to child abuse, chronic discrimination, oppression, marginalization, and toxic family dynamics.

RATES OF TRAUMA IN "SEVERE MENTAL ILLNESS"

A lot of times I'm in denial about the things that I do remember, 'cause I'm just like there's no way that something that horrible or that fantastical could have happened to me, it's just really hard to admit to … And I start telling my therapist things like "This can't be real, I must just be psychotic and making it up, and I'm delusional" because it just, it couldn't have happened that way. P3

I think it should be the goal of the therapist to have a space for hearing some horrific stuff. And some of that stuff, I know historically, can be really controversial, … I wonder if that's part of the reason why some of the leading trauma therapists want to just go away from the whole psychosis thing because it's almost a way to discredit somebody. P13

It was Pierre Janet, over a century ago, who first proclaimed widely that the medical establishment denied the existence of trauma and its effects, to the point of the establishment focusing too heavily on the biological domain (Janet, 1907/1965). By the time of the publication of the *DSM* in 1980, the women's rights movement and the political clout of the US military veterans had forced society, and, in turn, psychiatry, to recognize trauma and the resulting psychological effects more widely. (e.g., Middleton, 2013; Stern, 1996; van der Kolk, Brown, & van der Hart, 1989). Yet, the most recent version of the diagnostic bible (*DSM-5*; American Psychiatric Association, 2013) continues to separate recognized reactions to trauma from purported real *mental illness*, demonstrating just some of the ongoing ideological and political factions underlying the current paradigm.

It is commonly accepted that PTSD and dissociative disorders are associated with significant trauma. The very definition and diagnostic criteria for PTSD require an identifiable traumatic impetus for the subsequent distress. Although not as explicit, dissociative disorders are purposefully placed in proximity to the specific trauma disorders in the *DSM* to acknowledge their traumatic basis (American Psychiatric Association, 2013). Similarly, BPD is commonly accepted as being based in developmental trauma, with up to 80% to 90% reporting overt childhood trauma, such as sexual abuse (Herman, Perry, & Van der Kolk, 1989; Krause-Utz, Frost, Winter, & Elzinga, 2017; Mosquera & Steele, 2017). Yet, categories considered as representing illness or serious mental illness are separated out as being largely genetic or neurological, despite the accumulation of robust contrary evidence.

Non-affective psychosis (meaning the person is more shutdown emotionally than, say, psychotic depression) is more commonly diagnosed in economically deprived and socially isolated areas (Richardson, Hameed, Perez, Jones, & Kirkbride, 2017), as well as among men (Jongsma et al., 2018; Perez et al., 2016). Conversely, affective psychosis and "positive symptoms", such as paranoia, extrasensory perceptions, cognitive disorganization, and affect dysregulation, are more common among women

(Abel, Drake, & Goldstein, 2010; Castle, Wessely, & Murray, 1993; Cotton et al., 2009; Lindamer, Lohr, Harris, McAdams, & Jeste, 1999; Zhang et al., 2012) and are more closely associated with overt trauma, such as physical abuse (e.g., Read, Agar, Argyle, & Aderhold, 2003). This suggests that these differences lie along a continuum of emotional expression, at least partially along the lines of social acceptability for certain groups to be emotional. It is not coincidental, then, that DID tends to have a greater association with "positive symptoms", and is also almost primarily given to women (e.g., Hartung & Widiger, 1998), while schizophrenia, and its association with "negative symptoms", or withdrawal, apathy, and flat emotions, is more common among men, the economically disadvantaged, and minority racial groups (Abel et al., 2010; Aleman, Kahn, & Selten, 2003; Coleman et al., 2016; Feisthamel & Schwartz, 2009; Willhite et al., 2008).

Aside from gender and racial biases, the evidence supporting a specific and likely causal relationship between trauma and schizophrenia spectrum disorders is quite robust across varied cultures (Ayazi, Swartz, Eide, Lien, & Hauff, 2016; Honings et al., 2017; Mansueto & Faravelli, 2017; Matheson, Shepherd, Pinchbeck, Laurens, & Carr, 2013; McGrath et al., 2017; Morkved et al., 2017; Varese et al., 2012). Childhood adversity, such as bullying and child abuse, continues to be independently associated with risk of developing psychotic phenomena in both childhood (Arseneault et al., 2011) and adulthood (Ajnakina et al., 2016), independent of so-called genetic liability, IQ, and socioeconomic status. Bullying, specifically, has been shown to be directly related to paranoid thoughts and cognitive disorganization in twin studies (Singham et al., 2017). Being a minority immigrant (versus a White migrant) is specifically associated with increased risk of psychosis, independent of socioeconomic status (Kirkbride et al., 2017), while being Black in itself predicts a diagnosis of schizophrenia (Barnes, 2013; Feisthamel & Schwartz, 2009; Foulks, 2004).

There is also a dose-response relationship; the more severe the trauma, the higher the risk of psychosis or a diagnosis of schizophrenia (Cutajar et al., 2010; Janssen et al., 2004; McGrath et al., 2017), with those who have the most severe child abuse experiences at a 48 times (!) greater likelihood of developing psychosis than those without such adversity (Bentall, Wickham, Shevlin, & Varese, 2012). In addition to this cumulative effect, there also appears to be some specificity of certain adverse experiences (i.e., bullying) and specific psychotic phenomena (i.e., paranoia; Dvir,

Denietolis, & Frazier, 2013; Morkved et al., 2017). In fact, not only does childhood trauma and/or a diagnosis of PTSD predict psychotic phenomena (Kelleher et al., 2012; Powers, Fani, Cross, Ressler, & Bradley, 2016), but it has been suggested to be directly causal above and beyond any ostensible biological predispositions (Read, van Os, Morrison, & Ross, 2005; Shevlin et al., 2011; van Winkel, van Nierop, Myin-Germeys, & van Os, 2012).

Developmental trauma is also a major risk factor for later problems with emotional regulation and impulse control, leading to possible bipolar diagnoses (Aas et al., 2016). Children who have experienced childhood physical abuse are especially likely to have increased odds of later diagnoses of attention-deficit hyperactivity and bipolar disorders (Sugaya et al., 2012). Child abuse, in general, is associated with manic experiences (Levitan et al., 1998), as well as greater dysfunction and increased suicide attempts (Etain et al., 2013). In addition to overt abuse, parental loss and interpersonal trauma are significantly associated with a bipolar diagnosis (Mortensen, Pedersen, Melbye, Mors, & Ewald, 2003; Neria et al., 2008), while emotional abuse appears to have a particularly robust odds of leading to a bipolar diagnosis (Palmier-Claus, Berry, Bucci, Mansell, & Varese, 2016). Further, the drugs used for people who are diagnosed with depression are known to directly cause mania, leading to a major inflation in the number of diagnoses of bipolar disorder among trauma victims (e.g., Healy, 2012).

Unipolar depression is a common diagnosis among many with and without abuse, while those who get diagnosed with psychotic depression are most often those with a history of child abuse (Gaudiano & Zimmerman, 2010). Similar to non-affective psychosis, there is specificity and a dose-response relationship between childhood trauma and psychotic depression (van Dam et al., 2015). Additionally, people diagnosed with depression and who have histories of childhood trauma are also less likely to respond to standard interventions (Nanni, Uher, & Danese, 2012; Shamseddeen et al., 2011), often earning them the label of being "treatment resistant". Perhaps more important, the construct of depression is not universal (Summerfield, 2017) and is expressed differently among different cultures and ethnicities (Alang, 2016). This is an important point when considering that more severe illness categories are generally given to non-White, poorer, and immigrant populations, when in fact in some circumstances it could just be a different way of expressing the same internal experience.

In general, individuals labeled as having serious mental illness are significantly more likely to have experienced trauma, and more specifically, interpersonal trauma (Mauritz, Goossens, Draijer, & van Achterberg, 2013), than the general population. And, approximately one-third of these individuals also meet the full criteria for a trauma disorder (Mauritz et al., 2013). At the same time, those individuals who have a diagnosis of PTSD have an increased risk of later diagnoses of schizophrenia spectrum disorders and bipolar disorders, independent of familial risk (Okkels, Trabjerg, Arendt, & Pedersen, 2016). The trauma of involuntary treatment and diagnoses can lead to increased distress, alteration of voices and belief systems, and increased suicidality (Hjorthoj, Madsen, Agerbo, & Nordentoft, 2014; Large & Ryan, 2014), indicating that, for some, the treatment for severe mental illness may actually create the very problem it purports to fix.

One major problem in looking at "trauma" is that it ignores those chronic life experiences that do not meet some arbitrary threshold of being considered "bad enough" to be called trauma. Prior to the rise in power of the biomedical model, family dynamics and severe communication problems, such as gaslighting (being manipulated into doubting one's own reality), double binds (being trapped between two irreconcilable options), and enmeshed relationships (lack of physical and/or emotional boundaries), were considered by family therapists as pathognomonic of severe psychological distress, especially psychosis (e.g., Bateson, Jackson, Haley, & Weakland, 1956). Psychotic experiences, particularly paranoia, are often demonstrated to be associated with fearful attachment to caregivers (e.g., Pearce et al., 2017). Further, experiences such as subjective incidents of chronic discrimination (Wallace, Nazroo, & Becares, 2016), relative poverty (meaning being poor in a rich environment or country; Read, 2010), living in a deprived neighborhood (Bhavsar, Fusar-Poli, & McGuire, 2017), general social adversity (Longden & Read, 2016), and being an ethnic minority (Kirkbride et al., 2017; Perez et al., 2016) are all independently associated with later experiences of mental health difficulties, including psychosis. It is not always about overt abuse. People suffer for a myriad of reasons that can never be fully captured in reductionistic questionnaires or numerical rating systems.

In addition to the problem of ignoring or being unable to fully capture unrecognized forms of "trauma", there is the problem of underreporting and denial (Goodman, Rosenberg, Mueser, & Drake, 1997; Goodman et al., 1999). Child abuse victims are notorious for either denying or retracting accusations of abuse (Hegeman, 2009; Howell, 2011). Ignoring trauma and blaming the brain not only repeats oppressive forces of denial, it also leads to the person diagnosed as being perceived as less than human (Pavon & Vaes, 2017) and decreased empathy on the part of clinicians (Lebowitz & Ahn, 2014). In turn, placing the problem in the individual inadvertently perpetuates beliefs of helplessness, individual blame, and minimization of trauma (e.g., Goldsmith, Barlow, & Freyd, 2004). The mental illness paradigm provides an excellent scapegoat by offering an illusion of explanation for emotional distress without ever having to do the difficult work of examining family dynamics, involving social services, and/or disturbing the status quo (Bunston, Franich-Ray, & Tatlow, 2017; Longden, Read, & Dillon, 2016).

It has frequently been demonstrated that those who internalize a biomedical explanation for their difficulties tend to have a decreased sense of responsibility for their behaviors or less motivation to change (see Haslam, 2011 for a review). In addition to increased helplessness, by blaming the brain or genes, family dynamics and social adversity are easily ignored or minimized, by patients, clinicians, and society alike. Children wish to protect their parents and fear child services, and few people want to acknowledge the injustice and chaos of the world (see Lerner, 1980, for a discussion on the need to believe in a "just world"). The current mental health paradigm provides this illusion of order and justice, which, of course, is why it works so well as an ideology.

BIOLOGICAL PATTERNS CORRELATE WITH LIFE EXPERIENCE, NOT THE DSM

She calls it "non-organic mania", where I get manic symptoms but she doesn't think that it's from a bipolar cause ... I do have hallucinations and things like that, but she thinks that a lot of those hallucinations, visually and tactual and all the rest of it probably come from a trigger basis and that it looks very similar to bipolar and you treat it the same way as bipolar but it's not bipolar. P8

The 1990s saw a popular trend of psychiatry and pharmaceutical companies promoting the idea that mental illnesses were specific disorders caused by neurochemical imbalances in the brain that could specifically be targeted by psychoactive drugs. This was a profit-driven theory, promulgated originally by Pfizer, the makers of Prozac, and has since been demonstrated to be nothing more than a "myth" (Leo & Lacasse, 2008; Pies, 2011). In addition to the myth of chemical imbalances, psychiatric drugs also do not have any specific effect on DSM-defined disorders beyond general effects of numbing and sedating, nor is there any promotion of healthy brain growth associated with psychiatric drugs (Lakhan & Kirchgessner, 2012; Moncrieff, 2008, 2013). There also are no deteriorating or neurotoxic effects of psychosis (Ho et al., 2003; McGlashan, 2006), nor is there any protective function of antipsychotics on the brain (de Haan, van Der Gaag, & Wolthaus, 2000) despite proclamations otherwise. The Decade of the Brain, as the 1990s were designated by President George H. W. Bush, resulted in no clinical advances in psychiatry, and due to extraordinary methodological issues, the little bit of information that has arisen remains questionable at best (see, e.g., Venkatasubramanian & Keshavan, 2016).

What biological differences have been found in psychiatric populations are consistently shown to be associated with environmental factors, especially child abuse, rather than DSM-defined diagnoses or context-independent brain diseases. For instance, dopamine dysregulation is often suggested to be a pathway by which psychotic experiences develop, yet childhood trauma and social isolation alter brain areas associated with dopamine (Selten, Booij, Buwalda, & Meyer-Lindenberg, 2017). Genes and neurological pathways associated with inflammation are suggested to be potential causes of mania, psychosis, and depression (Barron, Hafizi, Andreazza, & Mizrahi, 2017; Sawa & Sedlak, 2016), yet inflammation is commonly known to be a direct result of chronic stress, social oppression, and trauma (Snyder-Mackler et al., 2016). Alterations in cortisol response are found in populations diagnosed with a psychotic disorder (Berger et al., 2016), yet cortisol is a hormone directly associated with the stress response. Child maltreatment is associated with decreased volume in brain areas associated with memory and decision-making (Selten et al., 2017; Teicher, Anderson, & Polcari, 2012), which also are areas commonly associated with a broad range of psychiatric disorders. This is not to say that understanding some of the biological pathways linking environmental injury to pain or emotional distress is unimportant; rather, to insinuate biological causation or reduction of complex emotions and behaviors to simple biological pathways is insulting and defeatist, nor does it indicate specificity of disease.

Despite almost half a century of looking for biological markers of mental illness, not a single one has been found for any diagnosis, even with the extraordinary bias and manipulations of language rife within this area of study (Prata, Mechelli, & Kapur, 2014). Psychological phenomena, such as hearing voices, show the same brain activity across diagnostic and nonclinical populations (Baumeister, Sedgwick, Howes, & Peters, 2017). Further, many of the brain abnormalities that have been purported to be evidence of brain disease have been found to actually be the result of chronic use of psychiatric drugs (e.g., Ho, Andreasen, Ziebell, Pierson, & Magnotta, 2011; Husa et al., 2014) and are non-specific to DSM-defined disorders.

In fact, most of the brain alterations demonstrated by brain scans are those that may be related to large parts of the brain, often associated with stress and fear, that become activated under certain conditions or in various states of mind, again with little difference between diagnoses (Sprooten et al., 2017). These alterations may also reflect the ways in which individuals make meaning out of their experiences, and so this subjective creation of reality may actually result in differing biological profiles rather than be caused by them (Cicchetti, 2002). Additionally, difference does not equate with disorder; for instance, individuals who have experienced childhood adversity tend to have problems in the prefrontal cortex and executive functioning (meaning they have problems with inhibitions and decision-making). Yet, being able to quickly shift attention in this way is adaptive in unpredictable environments (Mittal, Griskevicius, Simpson, Sung, & Young, 2015). In other words, differences in brain functioning do not equate with universal mental impairment and may, in fact, be associated with enhancements under specific circumstances (such as stressful and violent environments).

All of these brain studies, however, presuppose that there is an objective, normal brain that serves as a control to compare to. Yet, it appears as though much of the brain imaging research is biased along racial and socioeconomic lines, with White, highly educated, high socioeconomic status individuals serving as the "norm", despite demographic factors demonstrating drastically different brain pattern profiles (LeWinn, Sheridan, Keyes, Hamilton, & McLaughlin, 2017). Additionally, it has been estimated that up to 70% of these brain scan studies may actually be false positives, or have found significant results when there actually are none (Eklund, Nichols, & Knutsson, 2016). Even with all of this, a recent review by neuroscientists Holmes and Patrick (2018) provides evidence for the evolutionary necessity of variation in brain function, the fact that there is no "normal" brain demonstrating ideal functioning, and that there is no single optimum state to strive toward. It needs to be stated again that difference does not equal disease.

While these biological phenomena may mediate the process from psycho-logical trauma to specific psychic phenomena (e.g., Howes & McCutcheon, 2017) and are interesting from an academic perspective, it does not neces-sarily mean that the traumatic origin and psychosocial basis for these experi-ences should take a back seat to biological intervention and understanding. If the study of neuroscience in psychiatry is really more a study of the effects of stress, adversity, social isolation and oppression, and so on, then this should be exciting because preventative efforts can be enhanced now, instead of waiting for some promised day for a magic pill or technological invention that can miraculously make human suffering cease to exist.

GENETICS, EPIGENETICS, AND EUGENICS

[I] became quite concerned because I was getting very typical bipolar symp-toms—that's when I really started taking it seriously and trying to go to libraries and things in my spare time trying to figure out what it was, and starting to look into my family history. P8

The mental health field and the study of genetics have a sordid and unfortunate history embedded in harmful and discriminatory theories that contributed to eugenics and other great social harms.[1] Psychology, despite its many advances and positive influences, has also been central in discrimi-natory and elitist practices, beginning with its primary role in the eugenics movement (Black, 2003), to the oppression of Blacks and Native Americans (Hilton, 2011), and most recently, and perhaps notoriously, with its role in assisting illegal torture practices at Guantanamo Bay (see Hoffman et al., 2015). Jennifer Freyd, a psychologist specializing in trauma, has described these practices as a specific type of trauma called "institutional betrayal" (e.g., Gómez, Smith, Gobin, Tang, & Freyd, 2016).

Since the expansion of genetic research, a gene association and deter-ministic perspective of human behavior has been suggested for every-thing from suicidality (Shabalin et al., 2017) and neuroticism (Luciano et al., 2018) to years of schooling or education attainment (Domingue, Belsky, Conley, Harris, & Boardman, 2015), voting behaviors (Dawes & Fowler, 2009), food preferences (Eriksson et al., 2012; Liu et al., 2017), and even a fear of the dentist (Binkley et al., 2009). It is as if humans are essentially preprogrammed vessels operated blindly by all-powerful data sets passed down from generation to generation; there is rarely a vested interest in examining other reasons for statistical associations like, for instance, culture.

Genetics research may be promising for early intervention in areas such as Huntington's disease (Paulsen, 2010), which happens to be an entirely genetic disease. However, even with strongly genetically associated disorders, there still is no clinical usefulness to genetic testing beyond knowing one is at risk or already developing the disease (e.g., Muthane, 2011). In psychiatry, however, this research has proven futile, with the few positive associations found thus far having tiny statistical relationships with particular diagnoses across thousands of genetic loci and having absolutely zero clinical utility.[2]

The ongoing search for "missing heritability" is based on the assumption that psychiatric diagnoses, specifically schizophrenia, must be associated with specific genes due to the "high heritability" found from twin and adoption studies, but that these genes just still need to be found. Firstly, the term *heritability* is extremely misleading (Moore & Shenk, 2016); it is a statistical number that estimates the percentage of variation of certain traits (like, for instance, paranoid thinking) that is likely due to genetic factors. It does not represent how inheritable a trait is, nor does it provide information about the cause of a trait and the relative influence of genes or environment in the development of the trait, and has little actual value beyond the image it creates in one's mind when discussed.

Further, these estimates are based on twin studies of people who have been diagnosed with a particular disorder, namely, schizophrenia, and the overlap of identical twins (sharing 100% of genes) having the same diagnosis (*concordance*). Yet, these twin studies are based on biased and flawed methodology, relying on the assumption that identical twins do not experience more similar environments than non-identical (fraternal) twins. Even with these biased advantages, they still do not find that identical twins are concordant more than about half the time (and, sometimes, much less than that; Hilker et al., 2017).[3] Heritability has even been suggested to exist when no correlation or association was found at all between biological parents and offspring (Joseph, 2013).

The most recent twin study research concerning schizophrenia found that identical twins were concordant (meaning they both were considered positive for having schizophrenia) about 15% of the time (Hilker et al., 2017). Note that a true genetic disease, such as Huntington's disease, is one that finds 100% concordance between identical twins. Despite low identical twin concordance, twin researchers and psychiatry still perpetuate the conclusion that this "disease" is "highly heritable" with a "high genetic risk".

Although the evidence for the link between adversity and psychiatric diagnoses is robust, funding for ongoing research continues to almost exclusively be dedicated to neurological and genetic topics (Erlandsson & Punzi, 2016; Ioannidis, 2016; Joyner, Paneth, & Ioannidis, 2016). This is the case even considering the lack of there being a measurable effect on life improvement related to any of these described progressive advancements (Joyner et al., 2016). In addition to the lack of any measurable effect on improved clinical practice or understanding of psychological distress, genetic research is inconclusive, at best, and continues to lack support for the hypothesis that these are discrete disorders associated with specific genes.

Despite the assumed heritability of psychiatric diagnoses, there have not been any replicated identifications of specific genetic loci that can account for this (hence the idea of "missing heritability"; Bohacek, Gapp, Saab, & Mansuy, 2013). Even the most hardline proponents of the genetic model of psychiatric difficulties have acknowledged that the distribution of genetic risk for conditions such as schizophrenia is so wide that everyone carries some degree of risk (Kendler, 2015). The most commonly studied candidate genes for schizophrenia, assumed largely to be a "highly heritable" (e.g., Sullivan, Kendler, & Neale, 2003) disease, are no more associated with the diagnosis beyond chance (Edwards, Bacanu, Bigdeli, Moscati, & Kendler, 2016; Johnson et al., 2017) and do not replicate or predict vulnerability across various ethnic groups (Prasad et al., 2017; Vassos et al., 2017).

Genetic association studies' findings are generally highly inflated (Holland et al., 2017), contain numerous methodological errors (Rubanovich & Khromov-Borisov, 2016), are based on biased research designs and numerous flawed, faith-based assumptions (Charney, 2017), and are more the result of statistical artifact rather than any true effect (e.g., Fish, Capra, & Bush, 2016). Even with these biases and inflated results, the "breakthrough" studies rarely have findings that account for more than a tiny fraction of the population variance in risk for particular disorders, like schizophrenia (Levinson et al., 2012; Sekar et al., 2016) or bipolar disorder (Ikeda, Saito, Kondo, & Iwata, 2017). Overall, the genetic findings thus far have been useless in terms of developing clinical interventions or understanding emotional distress, similarly to diagnoses in general (e.g., Dubovsky, 2016).

On the other hand, epigenetics, or the study of how the environment impacts the expression of genes, is presumed to be an explanatory factor that both considers context (i.e., trauma) yet still adheres to the defective gene pool mentality (Teicher & Samson, 2013), sometimes requiring extraordinary mental gymnastics to do so (e.g., Diwadkar, Bustamante, Rai, & Uddin, 2014). In general, the idea is that the environment affects how genes are expressed and this environmental effect can alter genetic expression across generations (Moore, 2017). It is a term that represents a highly complex theoretical field of study and means different things to different people (Stelmach & Nerlich, 2015).

Many researchers and clinicians have argued that the fields of neurology and genetics too frequently ignore the effects of early childhood development and adversity (e.g., Greenberg, 2005), while expressing hope that these fields will soon realize the importance of context and environment (Ikeda et al., 2017). Stress and trauma have, indeed, been shown to alter genetic structure and to damage DNA (Dimitroglou et al., 2003). At the same time, patterns in families demonstrate reenactments from one generation to the next, often in addition to denial and lack of awareness (McCollum, 2015). In addition, previous epigenetic findings suggesting that changes in DNA can be passed on from one generation to the next may be entirely explained by lifestyle factors, such as smoking (see Marzi et al., 2018).

Focusing on the hypothetical genetic alterations of the environment, especially across generations, ignores the repeated trauma and adversity experienced in the here and now while averting responsibility to some unseen factor that may or may not actually even exist. Some have expressed concerns about the field of epigenetics representing a return to eugenics (Pickersgill, Niewöhner, Müller, Martin, & Cunningham-Burley, 2013) and a metaphoric "intergenerational blame-game" (Stelmach & Nerlich, 2015) wherein people no longer need to be concerned about their own behaviors, but rather blame generations prior for passing down bad genes due to their (or their society's) problematic behaviors and lifestyles. Not only does it run the risk of contributing once again to absolution of responsibility, but, perhaps more dangerously, genetic explanations of so-called mental illness are consistently associated with harsher and more dehumanized treatments, decreased hope, and more extreme forms of biological interventions (e.g., Phelan, Yang, & Cruz-Rojas, 2006).

While surely there is some variation in any individual's biological and genetic make-up at birth, and everyone is more or less susceptible to temperamental adaptations across the lifespan, the evidence consistently demonstrates the effects of lifestyle and environment on biological expression. For instance, inflammation, and biological and genetic mechanisms associated with the immune response and inflammation, are linked with and may even play a mediating role in the development of emotional distress, including psychosis (Baumeister, Akhtar, Ciufolini, Pariante, & Mondelli, 2016). However, this immune response is not just a biological mishap unrelated to context; rather, childhood adversity contributes to an enduring inflammatory response, similar to that seen with physical wounds (Danese & Baldwin, 2017), and even has specific profiles associated with specific types of trauma (Baumeister et al., 2016).

Perhaps more importantly, mindfulness and other mind-body interventions actually reverse the genetic expression involved in the inflammatory response (Buric, Farias, Jong, Mee, & Brazil, 2017)! Similarly, what is being tested when looking at genetics is not even clear: what is the "predisposition" that is considered? Is it for a purported psychiatric disease triggered by abuse and oppression? Or, perhaps, might it be a particular sensitivity to the environment (which, ironically, is considered to actually be favored by natural selection; Cheong, Tan, Xie, & Jones, 2016)? In the end, regardless of purported associations of genetic variation and so-called serious mental illness, these associations, at best, remain very small, while there is consistently a medium to large effect found for childhood adversity (e.g., Matheson et al., 2013).

Difference does not equate with objective value judgments of disease or defect. A genetic vulnerability to, say, experiencing voice-hearing or mania in response to adversity versus, say, an apathetic and dismissive perception of individuals deemed to be inferior to one's self is surely variable throughout the population. To insinuate or extrapolate, however, that one form of response is diseased while the other is not only acceptable but admirable (see leaders in politics, finance, or corporations, for instance) is a leap of logic based in ideology, not science. Even considering that there is, in fact, some small inherited vulnerability to later emotional distress, it still requires environmental injury to be "triggered" in the first place.

LIFESTYLE AND RELATIONSHIPS MATTER

And what I discovered was that massive amounts of healing don't happen in therapy and it certainly doesn't happen in isolation, it happens in engaging life. P5

I feel better when I do exercise, so I exercise, and that's helpful ... I try to take care of my physical body too, as much as I'm able, cause it helps me feel better about myself, and if I feel physically, that's very helpful with my emotional and my mental health too I've found, personally. P6

As stated by the Special Rapporteur on Torture and Other Cruel, Inhuman or Degrading Treatment or Punishment of the United Nations: "The excessive use of medications and other biomedical interventions, based on a reductive neurobiological paradigm causes more harm than good, undermines the right to health, and must be abandoned" (Mendez, 2013). The focus on biological defect and diseases of the brain lends itself to a primarily biological treatment framework. Even if acknowledging the adversity-based etiology of psychological distress, there still are those who will focus on the diseased brain or genetic alterations that require biological intervention or render the person helpless. While psychiatric drugs can be helpful for some (as can any kind of drug!), this does not necessarily mean that these drugs alter biology in a healthy way, nor that they are always necessary. In fact, it turns out that lifestyle and relationships are much more likely to lead to healthy alterations in biology than any invention based on technology or chemistry.

Psychotherapy has been demonstrated to alter brain functioning (Mason, Peters, Williams, & Kumari, 2017) as well as result in changes in genes associated with the stress response (Roberts et al., 2014, 2015). In fact, brain alterations after psychotherapy can predict higher subjective ratings of recovery for people diagnosed with a psychotic disorder over eight years later (Mason et al., 2017). Changes in social standing have been shown to alter immune functioning at the genetic and cellular levels in primates (Snyder-Mackler et al., 2016). In other words, empowerment can actually change genetic expression. Helping others also has been shown to decrease stress-induced inflammation and health problems (Poulin & Holman, 2013). Meditation and other mind-body interventions have additionally been shown to have an effect on gene expression and a reduction in inflammatory reactions induced by stress (Buric et al., 2017). Developing relationships, empowerment, helping others and attending to the physical body all demonstrate powerful effects on the brain, genetic expression, and inflammation—these also happen to some of the primary components that people find to be helpful in the recovery process.

There is a place for professional intervention, such as psychotherapy, for some, and psychoactive drugs that help avert acute crises. However, the idea that these interventions are somehow superior to lifestyle changes, relationships, or non-technical approaches like yoga is an idea that is solely based on ideology and vested interests in maintaining professional standing and power. It is not based in science, and, in fact, may actually defy it. People are different, and difference from the dominating norm is not necessarily evidence of inferiority or disease. Further, trauma, oppression, and adversity are a part of life, whether we wish to acknowledge or appreciate it or not. And, long-term healing happens through changes in the environment; changes that have been common sense for centuries prior to the advent of industrialization. Relationships matter. Relaxation matters. Nutrition matters. Hope and purpose matter. Nature matters. Love matters.

NOTES

1. See Black (2003) for an in-depth academic exploration of this history. In his book *War Against the Weak*, Black details how the early efforts to cleanse society of its supposed unfit and undesirable were directly associated with the development of intelligence testing, judicial and bureaucratic rules guiding the mental health system, the development of the ideology of scientism, much of psychological practices and beliefs, social engineering, and Nazi ideology. After the tragedy of the Holocaust, eugenics fell out of favor for obvious reasons and thus needed rebranding. After World War II, eugenics became transformed into the study of genetics. This new field of academics supported the power of the elite, with undesirable human qualities such as poverty, particular racial groups, personality traits, criminality, and non-conformity being asserted as hereditary and existing within inferior familial stock. These theories and values continue to infiltrate much of mental health practices, have long been supported by the veneer of science, and promote racist, discriminatory, and oppressive practices whether intentional or not.

2. See Dubovsky (2016) for a summary overview. In this editorial, Dubovsky discusses the many purported findings in psychiatric genetics research and the numerous problems, including the larger problem with descriptive diagnoses, the difficulty (if not impossibility) of separating environmental effects on genes from pure genetic effects, the small effect across thousands of genetic loci found, the lack of clinical utility, and the more generalized link between specific experiences (i.e., inflammation) and genetic alterations versus those associated specifically with DSM-defined diagnoses. See also Whitaker (2010), Bentall (2009), and, especially, Ross and Pam (1995) for in-depth discussions on the problems in psychiatric genetics research, the lack of replicable, useful findings, and the ideology that drives the ongoing funding of this research despite little support for its continuation.

3. Jay Joseph has dedicated much of his career to breaking down these twin studies and the problems of genetic explanations of schizophrenia. His most recent book *Schizophrenia and Genetics: The End of an Illusion* provides an up-to-date exploration and overview of the methodological flaws, biases, and environmental confounds in schizophrenia family, twin, and adoption studies. He shows that genetic researchers usually fail to consider that their hypotheses may be incorrect despite decades of evidence suggesting that they likely are, and he calls for a focus on environmental and non-medical approaches.

REFERENCES

Aas, M., Henry, C., Andreassen, O. A., Bellivier, F., Melle, I., & Etain, B. (2016). The role of childhood trauma in bipolar disorders. [journal article]. *International Journal of Bipolar Disorders, 4*(1), 2. https://doi.org/10.1186/s40345-015-0042-0

Abel, K. M., Drake, R., & Goldstein, J. M. (2010). Sex differences in schizophrenia. *International Review of Psychiatry, 22*(5), 417–428.

Ajnakina, O., Trotta, A., Oakley-Hannibal, E., Di Forti, M., Stilo, S. A., Kolliakou, A., ... Fisher, H. L. (2016). Impact of childhood adversities on specific symptom dimensions in first-episode psychosis. *Psychological Medicine, 46*(2), 317–326. https://doi.org/10.1017/s0033291715001816

Alang, S. M. (2016). "Black folk don't get no severe depression": Meanings and expressions of depression in a predominantly black urban neighborhood in Midwestern United States. *Social Science & Medicine, 157*, 1–8.

Aleman, A., Kahn, R. S., & Selten, J. P. (2003). Sex differences in the risk of schizophrenia: Evidence from meta-analysis. *Archives of General Psychiatry, 60*(6), 565–571.

American Psychiatric Association. (2013). *Diagnostic and statistical manual of mental disorders: DSM-5.* Washington, DC: American Psychiatric Association.

Arseneault, L., Cannon, M., Fisher, H. L., Polanczyk, G., Moffitt, T. E., & Caspi, A. (2011). Childhood trauma and children's emerging psychotic symptoms: A genetically sensitive longitudinal cohort study. *American Journal of Psychiatry, 168*(1), 65–72.

Ayazi, T., Swartz, L., Eide, A. H., Lien, L., & Hauff, E. (2016). Psychotic-like experiences in a conflict-affected population: A cross-sectional study in South Sudan. *Social Psychiatry and Psychiatric Epidemiology, 51*(7), 971–979.

Barnes, A. (2013). Race and schizophrenia in four types of hospitals. *Journal of Black Studies, 44*(6), 665–681.

Barron, H., Hafizi, S., Andreazza, A. C., & Mizrahi, R. (2017). Neuroinflammation and oxidative stress in psychosis and psychosis risk. *International Journal of Molecular Sciences, 18*(3), 651. https://doi.org/10.3390/ijms18030651

Bateson, G., Jackson, D. D., Haley, J., & Weakland, J. (1956). Toward a theory of schizophrenia. *Behavioral Science, 1*(4), 251–264.

Baumeister, D., Akhtar, R., Ciufolini, S., Pariante, C. M., & Mondelli, V. (2016). Childhood trauma and adulthood inflammation: A meta-analysis of peripheral C-reactive protein, interleukin-6 and tumour necrosis factor-alpha. *Molecular Psychiatry, 21*(5), 642–649. https://doi.org/10.1038/mp.2015.67

Baumeister, D., Sedgwick, O., Howes, O., & Peters, E. (2017). Auditory verbal hallucinations and continuum models of psychosis: A systematic review of the healthy voice-hearer literature. *Clinical Psychology Review, 51*, 125–141.

Bentall, R. P. (2009). *Doctoring the mind.* New York, NY: New York University Press.

Bentall, R. P., Wickham, S., Shevlin, M., & Varese, F. (2012). Do specific early-life adversities lead to specific symptoms of psychosis? A study. *Schizophrenia Bulletin, 38*, 734–740.

Berger, M., Kraeuter, A. K., Romanik, D., Malouf, P., Amminger, G. P., & Sarnyai, Z. (2016). Cortisol awakening response in patients with psychosis: Systematic review and meta-analysis. *Neuroscience & Biobehavioral Reviews, 68*, 157–166.

Bhavsar, V., Fusar-Poli, P., & McGuire, P. (2017). Neighbourhood deprivation is positively associated with detection of the ultra-high risk (UHR) state for psychosis in South East London. *Schizophrenia Research, 8*(17), 30334–30331. https://doi.org/10.1016/j.schres.2017.06.00

Binkley, C. J., Beacham, A., Neace, W., Gregg, R. G., Liem, E. B., & Sessler, D. I. (2009). Genetic variations associated with red hair color and fear of dental pain, anxiety regarding dental care and avoidance of dental care. *Journal of the American Dental Association (1939), 140*(7), 896–905.

Black, E. (2003). *War against the weak: Eugenics and America's campaign to create a master race.* Washington, DC: Dialog Press.

Bohacek, J., Gapp, K., Saab, B. J., & Mansuy, I. M. (2013). Transgenerational epigenetic effects on brain functions. *Biological Psychiatry, 73*(4), 313–320.

Bunston, W., Franich-Ray, C., & Tatlow, S. (2017). A diagnosis of denial: How mental health classification systems have struggled to recognise family violence as a serious risk factor in the development of mental health issues for infants, children, adolescents, and adults. *Brain Sciences, 7*(133). https://doi.org/10.3390/brainsci7100133

Buric, I., Farias, M., Jong, J., Mee, C., & Brazil, I. A. (2017). What is the molecular signature of mind-body interventions? A systematic review of gene expression changes induced by meditation and related practices. *Frontiers in Immunology, 8*(670). https://doi.org/10.3389/fimmu.2017.00670

Castle, D. J., Wessely, S., & Murray, R. M. (1993). Sex and schizophrenia: Effects of diagnostic stringency, and associations with premorbid variables. *British Journal of Psychiatry, 162*, 658–664.

Charney, E. (2017). Genes, behavior, and behavior genetics. *Wiley Interdisciplinary Reviews: Cognitive Science, 8*(1–2), e1405–e1n/a. https://doi.org/10.1002/wcs.1405

Cheong, K. H., Tan, Z. X., Xie, N.-G., & Jones, M. C. (2016). A paradoxical evolutionary mechanism in stochastically switching environments. *Scientific Reports, 6*(34889). https://doi.org/10.1038/srep34889

Cicchetti, D. (2002). The impact of social experience on neurobiological systems: Illustration from a constructivist view of child maltreatment. *Cognitive Development, 17*, 1407–1428.

Coleman, K. J., Stewart, C., Waitzfelder, B. E., Zeber, J. E., Morales, L. S., Ahmed, A. T., … Simon, G. E. (2016). Racial-ethnic differences in psychiatric diagnoses and treatment across 11 health care systems in the mental health research network. *Psychiatric Services, 67*(7), 749–757.

Cotton, S. M., Lambert, M., Schimmelmann, B. G., Foley, D. L., Morley, K. L., McGorry, P. D., & Conus, P. (2009). Gender differences in premorbid, entry, treatment, and outcome characteristics in a treated epidemiological sample of 661 patients with first episode psychosis. *Schizophrenia Research, 114,* 17–24.

Cutajar, M. C., Mullen, P. E., Ogloff, J. R., Thomas, S. D., Wells, D. L., & Spataro, J. (2010). Schizophrenia and other psychotic disorders in a cohort of sexually abused children. *Archives of General Psychiatry, 67*(11), 1114–1119.

Danese, A., & Baldwin, J. R. (2017). Hidden wounds? Inflammatory links between childhood trauma and psychopathology. *Annual Review of Psychology, 68,* 517–544.

Dawes, C. T., & Fowler, J. H. (2009). Partisanship, Voting, and the Dopamine D2 Receptor Gene. *The Journal of Politics, 71*(3), 1157–1171. https://doi.org/10.1017/s002238160909094x

de Haan, L., van Der Gaag, M., & Wolthaus, J. (2000). Duration of untreated psychosis and the long-term course of schizophrenia. *European Psychiatry, 15*(4), 264–267.

Dimitroglou, E., Zafiropoulou, M., Messini-Nikolaki, N., Doudounakis, S., Tsilimigaki, S., & Piperakis, S. M. (2003). DNA damage in a human population affected by chronic psychogenic stress. *International Journal of Hygiene and Environmental Health, 206*(1), 39–44.

Diwadkar, V. A., Bustamante, A., Rai, H., & Uddin, M. (2014). Epigenetics, stress, and their potential impact on brain network function: A focus on the schizophrenia diatheses. *Frontiers in Psychiatry, 5,* 71. https://doi.org/10.3389/fpsyt.2014.00071

Domingue, B. W., Belsky, D. W., Conley, D., Harris, K. M., & Boardman, J. D. (2015). Polygenic influence on educational attainment: New evidence from the national longitudinal study of adolescent to adult health. *AERA Open, 1*(3). https://doi.org/10.1177/2332858415599972

Dubovsky, S. L. (2016). The limitations of genetic testing in psychiatry. [Editorial]. *Psychotherapy and Psychosomatics, 85,* 129–135.

Duran, E., Firehammer, J., & Gonzalez, J. (2008). Liberation psychology as the path toward healing cultural soul wounds. *Journal of Counseling & Development, 86*(3), 288–295.

Dvir, Y., Denietolis, B., & Frazier, J. A. (2013). Childhood trauma and psychosis. *Child and Adolescent Psychiatric Clinics of North America, 22*(4), 629–641.

Edwards, A. C., Bacanu, S. A., Bigdeli, T. B., Moscati, A., & Kendler, K. S. (2016). Evaluating the dopamine hypothesis of schizophrenia in a large-scale genome-wide association study. *Schizophrenia Research, 176,* 136–140.

Eklund, A., Nichols, T. E., & Knutsson, H. (2016). Cluster failure: Why fMRI inferences for spatial extent have inflated false-positive rates. *PNAS, 113,* 7900–7905.

Eriksson, N., Wu, S., Do, C. B., Kiefer, A. K., Tung, J. Y., Mountain, J. L., … Francke, U. (2012). A genetic variant near olfactory receptor genes influences cilantro preference. *Flavour, 1*(22). Retrieved from https://flavourjournal. biomedcentral.com/articles/10.1186/2044-7248-1-22;   https://doi.org/ 10.1186/2044-7248-1-22

Erlandsson, S., & Punzi, E. (2016). Challenging the ADHD consensus. *International Journal of Qualitative Studies on Health and Well-being, 11.* https://doi.org/10.3402/qhw.v11.31124

Etain, B., Aas, M., Andreassen, O. A., Lorentzen, S., Dieset, I., Gard, S., ... Henry, C. (2013). Childhood trauma is associated with severe clinical characteristics of bipolar disorders. *The Journal of Clinical Psychiatry, 74.* https://doi.org/10.4088/JCP.13m08353

Feisthamel, K. P., & Schwartz, R. C. (2009). Differences in mental health counselors' diagnoses based on client race: An investigation of adjustment, childhood, and substance-related disorders. *Journal of Mental Health Counseling, 31*(10), 47–59.

Fish, A. E., Capra, J. A., & Bush, W. S. (2016). Are interactions between cis-regulatory variants evidence for biological epistasis or statistical artifacts? *American Journal of Human Genetics, 99*(4), 817–830.

Foulks, E. F. (2004, April 15). Cultural variables in psychiatry. *Psychiatric Times, 21,* 28–29.

Gaudiano, B. A., & Zimmerman, M. (2010). The relationship between childhood trauma history and the psychotic subtype of major depression. *Acta Psychiatrica Scandinavica, 121*(6), 462–470.

Goldsmith, R. E., Barlow, M. R., & Freyd, J. J. (2004). Knowing and not knowing about trauma: Implications for therapy. *Psychotherapy: Theory, Research, Practice, Training, 41*(4), 448–463.

Gómez, J. M., Smith, C. P., Gobin, R. L., Tang, S. S., & Freyd, J. J. (2016). Collusion, torture, and inequality: Understanding the actions of the American Psychological Association as institutional betrayal. *Journal of Trauma & Dissociation, 17*(5), 527–544. https://doi.org/10.1080/15299732.2016.12 14436

Goodman, L., Rosenberg, S. D., Mueser, K. T., & Drake, R. (1997). Physical and sexual assault history in women with serious mental illness: Prevalence, correlates, treatment, and future research directions. *Schizophrenia Bulletin, 23*(4), 685–696.

Goodman, L., Thompson, K. M., Weinfurt, K., Corl, S., Acker, P., Mueser, K. T., & Rosenberg, S. D. (1999). Reliability of reports of violent victimization and posttraumatic stress disorder among men and women with serious mental illness. *Journal of Traumatic Stress, 12*(4), 587–599.

Greenberg, G. (2005). The limitations of behavior-genetic analyses: Comment on McGue, Elkins, Walden, and Iacono. *Developmental Psychology, 41*(6), 989–992.

Hartung, C. M., & Widiger, T. A. (1998). Gender differences in the diagnosis of mental disorders: Conclusions and controversies of the DSM-IV. *Psychological Bulletin, 123*(3), 260–278.

Haslam, N. (2011). Genetic essentialism, neuroessentialism, and stigma: Commentary on Dar-Nimrod and Heine. *Psychological Bulletin, 137*(5), 819–824. https://doi.org/10.1037/a0022386

Healy, D. (2012). *Pharmageddon*. Los Angeles, CA: University of California Press.

Hegeman, E. (2009). One or many? Commentary on paper by Debra Rothschild. *Psychoanalytic Dialogues, 19*, 188–196.

Herman, J., Perry, J. C., & Van der Kolk, B. A. (1989). Childhood trauma in borderline personality disorder. *American Journal of Psychiatry, 146*(4), 490–495.

Hilker, R., Helenius, D., Fagerlund, B., Skytthe, A., Christensen, K., Werge, T. M., … Glenthoj, B. (2017). Heritability of schizophrenia and schizophrenia spectrum based on the nationwide danish twin register. *Biological Psychiatry, 1*(17), 31905–31904.

Hilton, B. T. (2011). Frantz Fanon and colonialism: A psychology of oppression. *Journal of Scientific Psychology*, 45–59 Retrieved from http://www.psyencelab.com/uploads/5/4/6/5/54658091/frantz_fanon_and_colonialism.pdf

Hjorthoj, C. R., Madsen, T., Agerbo, E., & Nordentoft, M. (2014). Risk of suicide according to level of psychiatric treatment: A nationwide nested case-control study. *Social Psychiatry and Psychiatric Epidemiology, 49*, 1357–1365.

Ho, B. C., Alicata, D., Ward, J., Moser, D. J., O'Leary, D. S., Arndt, S., & Andreasen, N. C. (2003). Untreated initial psychosis: Relation to cognitive deficits and brain morphology in first-episode schizophrenia. *American Journal of Psychiatry, 160*(1), 142–148.

Ho, B. C., Andreasen, N. C., Ziebell, S., Pierson, R., & Magnotta, V. (2011). Long-term antipsychotic treatment and brain volumes. *Archives of General Psychiatry, 68*(2), 128–137.

Hoffman, D. H., Carter, D. J., Viglucci Lopez, C. R., Benzmiller, H. L., Guo, A. X., Yasir Latifi, S., & Craig, D. C. (2015). Report to the special committee of the board of directors of the American Psychological Association: Independent review relating to APA ethics guidelines, national security interrogations, and torture—Revised September 4, 2015. Retrieved from http://www.apa.org/independent-review/revised-report.pdf

Holland, D., Fan, C.-C., Frei, O., Shadrin, A. A., Smeland, O. B., Sundar, V. S., … Dale, A. M. (2017). Estimating inflation in GWAS summary statistics due to variance distortion from cryptic relatedness. *bioRxiv*. https://doi.org/10.1101/164939

Holmes, A. J., & Patrick, L. M. (2018). The myth of optimality in clinical neuroscience. *Trends in Cognitive Sciences, 22*(3), 241–257. https://doi.org/10.1016/j.tics.2017.12.006

Honings, S., Drukker, M., Ten Have, M., de Graaf, R., van Dorsselaer, S., & van Os, J. (2017). The interplay of psychosis and victimisation across the life course: A prospective study in the general population. *Social Psychiatry and Psychiatric Epidemiology, 52*(11), 1363–1374.

Howell, E. (2011). *Understanding and treating dissociative identity disorder: A relational approach.* New York, NY: Taylor and Francis Group, LLC.

Howes, O. D., & McCutcheon, R. (2017). Inflammation and the neural diathesis-stress hypothesis of schizophrenia: a reconceptualization. [Review]. *Translational Psychiatry, 7,* e1024. https://doi.org/10.1038/tp.2016.278 https://www.nature.com/articles/tp2016278#supplementary-information

Husa, A. P., Rannikko, I., Moilanen, J., Haapea, M., Murray, G. K., Barnett, J., ... Jaaskelainen, E. (2014). Lifetime use of antipsychotic medication and its relation to change of verbal learning and memory in midlife schizophrenia – An observational 9-year follow-up study. *Schizophrenia Research, 158*(1-3), 134–141.

Ikeda, M., Saito, T., Kondo, K., & Iwata, N. (2017). Genome-wide association studies of bipolar disorder: A systematic review of recent findings and their clinical implications. *Psychiatry and Clinical Neuroscience, 23*(10), 12611.

Ioannidis, J. P. A. (2016). Evidence-based medicine has been hijacked: A report to David Sackett. *Journal of Clinical Epidemiology, 73,* 82–86.

Janet, P. (1907/1965). *The major symptoms of hysteria.* New York: Hafner Publishing Company.

Janssen, I., Krabbendam, L., Bak, M., Hanssen, M., Vollebergh, W., De Graff, R., & van Os, J. (2004). Childhood abuse as a risk factor for psychotic experiences. *Acta Psychiatrica Scandinavica, 109,* 38–45.

Johnson, E. C., Border, R., Melroy-Greif, W. E., de Leeuw, C. A., Ehringer, M. A., & Keller, M. C. (2017). No evidence that schizophrenia candidate genes are more associated with schizophrenia than noncandidate genes. *Biological Psychiatry, 82*(10), 702–708. https://doi.org/10.1016/j.biopsych.2017.06.033

Jongsma, H. E., Gayer-Anderson, C., Lasalvia, A., Quattrone, D., Mule, A., Szoke, A., ... Kirkbride, J. B. (2018). Treated incidence of psychotic disorders in the multinational EU-GEI study. *JAMA Psychiatry, 75*(1), 36–46.

Joseph, J. (2013). The lost study: A 1998 adoption study of personality that found no genetic relationship between birthparents and their 240 adopted-away biological offspring. In R. M. Lerner & J. B. Benson (Eds.), *Embodiment and epigenesist: Theoretical and methodological issues in understanding the role of biology within the relational developmental system Part B: Ontogenetic dimensions* (pp. 93–124). New York: Elsevier Inc./Academic Press.

Joyner, M. J., Paneth, N., & Ioannidis, J. P. A. (2016). What happens when underperforming big ideas in research become entrenched? *JAMA, 316*(13), 1355–1356.

Kelleher, I., Keeley, H., Corcoran, P., Ramsay, H., Wasserman, C., Carli, V., ... Cannon, M. (2012). Childhood trauma and psychosis in a prospective cohort study: Cause, effect, and directionality. *American Journal of Psychiatry, 170*(7), 734–741.

Kendler, K. S. (2015). A joint history of the nature of genetic variation and the nature of schizophrenia. *Molecular Psychiatry, 20*(1), 77–83.

Kirkbride, J. B., Hameed, Y., Ioannidis, K., Ankireddypalli, G., Crane, C. M., Nasir, M., … Jones, P. B. (2017). Ethnic minority status, age-at-immigration and psychosis risk in rural environments: Evidence form the SEPEA Study. *Schizophrenia Bulletin.* https://doi.org/10.1093/schbul/sbx010

Krause-Utz, A., Frost, R., Winter, D., & Elzinga, B. M. (2017). Dissociation and alterations in brain function and structure: Implications for borderline personality disorder. *Current Psychiatry Reports, 19*(1), 6. https://doi.org/10.1007/s11920-017-0757-y

Lakhan, S. E., & Kirchgessner, A. (2012). Prescription stimulants in individuals with and without attention deficit hyperactivity disorder: Misuse, cognitive impact, and adverse effects. *Brain and Behavior, 2*(5), 661–677.

Large, M., & Ryan, C. J. (2014). Disturbing findings about the risk of suicide and psychiatric hospitals. *Journal of Social Psychiatry and Psychiatric Epidemiology, 40*(9), 1353–1355.

Lebowitz, M. S., & Ahn, W.-K. (2014). Effects of biological explanations for mental disorders on clinicians' empathy. *Proceedings of the National Academy of Sciences of the United States of America, 111*(50), 17786–17790. https://doi.org/10.1073/pnas.1414058111

Leo, J., & Lacasse, J. (2008). The media and the chemical imbalance theory of depression. *Society, 45*(1), 35–45.

Lerner, M. J. (1980). The belief in a just world. In *The belief in a just world: Perspectives in social psychology.* Boston, MA: Springer.

Levinson, D. F., Shi, J., Wang, K., Oh, S., Riley, B., Pulver, A. E., … Holmans, P. A. (2012). Genome-wide association study of multiplex schizophrenia pedigrees. *American Journal of Psychiatry, 169*(9), 963–973.

Levitan, R. D., Parikh, S. V., Lesage, A. D., Hegadoren, K. M., Adams, M., Kennedy, S. H., & Goering, P. N. (1998). Major depression in individuals with a history of childhood physical or sexual abuse: Relationship to neurovegetative features, mania, and gender. *American Journal of Psychiatry, 155*, 1746–1752.

LeWinn, K. Z., Sheridan, M. A., Keyes, K. M., Hamilton, A., & McLaughlin, K. A. (2017). Sample composition alters associations between age and brain structure. *Nature Communications, 8*(1), 874. https://doi.org/10.1038/s41467-017-00908-7

Lindamer, L. A., Lohr, J. B., Harris, M. J., McAdams, L. A., & Jeste, D. V. (1999). Gender-related clinical differences in older patients with schizophrenia. *Journal of Clinical Psychiatry, 60*(1), 61–67.

Liu, X.-p., Gao, B.-z., Han, F.-q., Fang, Z.-y., Yang, L.-m., Zhuang, M., … Zhang, Y.-y. (2017). Genetics and fine mapping of a purple leaf gene, BoPr, in ornamental kale (Brassica oleracea L. var. acephala). *BMC Genomics, 18*, 230. https://doi.org/10.1186/s12864-017-3613-x

Longden, E., & Read, J. (2016). Social adversity in the etiology of psychosis: A review of the evidence. *American Journal of Psychotherapy, 70,* 5–33.

Longden, E., Read, J., & Dillon, J. (2016). Improving community mental health services: The need for a paradigm shift. *The Israel Journal of Psychiatry and Related Sciences, 53*(1), 22–30.

Luciano, M., Hagenaars, S. P., Davies, G., David Hill, W., Clarke, T.-K., Shirali, M., … Deary, I. J. (2018). Association analysis in over 329,000 individuals identifies 116 independent variants influencing neuroticism. *Nature Genetics, 50*(1), 6–11. https://doi.org/10.1038/s41588-017-0013-8

Mansueto, G., & Faravelli, C. (2017). Recent life events and psychosis: The role of childhood adversities. *Psychiatry Research, 256,* 111–117.

Marzi, S. J., Sugden, K., Arseneault, L., Belsky, D. W., Burrage, J., Corcoran, D. L., … Caspi, A. (2018). Analysis of DNA methylation in young people: Limited evidence for an association between victimization stress and epigenetic variation in blood. *American Journal of Psychiatry.* https://doi.org/10.1176/appi.ajp.2017.17060693

Mason, L., Peters, E., Williams, S. C., & Kumari, V. (2017). Brain connectivity changes occurring following cognitive behavioural therapy for psychosis predict long-term recovery. *Translational Psychiatry, 7*(e1001). https://doi.org/10.1038/tp.2016.263

Matheson, S. L., Shepherd, A. M., Pinchbeck, R. M., Laurens, K. R., & Carr, V. J. (2013). Childhood adversity in schizophrenia: A systematic meta-analysis. *Psychological Medicine, 43*(2), 225–238.

Mauritz, M. W., Goossens, P. J. J., Draijer, N., & van Achterberg, T. (2013). Prevalence of interpersonal trauma exposure and trauma-related disorders in severe mental illness. *European Journal of Psychotraumatology, 4*(1), 19985. https://doi.org/10.3402/ejpt.v4i0.19985

McCollum, S. E. (2015). Multigenerational dissociation: A framework for building narrative. *Journal of Trauma & Dissociation, 16*(5), 563–576.

McGlashan, T. H. (2006). Is active psychosis neurotoxic? *Schizophrenia Bulletin, 32*(4), 609–613.

McGrath, J. J., Saha, S., Lim, C. C. W., Aguilar-Gaxiola, S., Alonso, J., Andrade, L. H., … Kessler, R. C. (2017). Trauma and psychotic experiences: transnational data from the World Mental Health Survey. *The British Journal of Psychiatry.* https://doi.org/10.1192/bjp.bp.117.205955

Mendez, J. E. (2013, March). Special Rapporteur on torture and other cruel, inhuman or degrading treatment or punishment. 22nd session of the Human Rights Council, Agenda Item 3, Geneva.

Middleton, W. (2013). Ongoing incestuous abuse during adulthood. *Journal of Trauma & Dissociation, 14,* 251–272.

Mittal, C., Griskevicius, V., Simpson, J. A., Sung, S., & Young, E. S. (2015). Cognitive adaptations to stressful environments: When childhood adversity enhances adult executive function. *Journal of Personality and Social Psychology,* *109*(4), 604–621.

Moncrieff, J. (2008). *The myth of the chemical cure: A critique of psychiatric drug treatment.* Basingstoke: Palgrave Macmillan.

Moncrieff, J. (2013). *The bitterest pills: The troubling story of antipsychotic drugs.* Basingstoke: Palgrave Macmillan.

Moore, D. S. (2017). Behavioral epigenetics. *Wiley Interdisciplinary Reviews: Systems Biology and Medicine, 9*(1), e1333–e1n/a. https://doi.org/10.1002/wsbm.1333

Moore, D. S., & Shenk, D. (2016). The heritability fallacy. *WIREs Cognitive Science.* https://doi.org/10.1002/wcs.1400

Morkved, N., Endsjo, M., Winje, D., Johnsen, E., Dovran, A., Arefjord, K., … Loberg, E. M. (2017). Childhood trauma in schizophrenia spectrum disorder as compared to other mental health disorders. *Psychosis, 9*(1), 48–56.

Mortensen, P. B., Pedersen, C. B., Melbye, M., Mors, O., & Ewald, H. (2003). Major depression in individuals with a history of childhood physical or sexual abuse: Relationship to neurovegetative features, mania, and gender. *Archives of General Psychiatry, 60,* 1209–1215.

Mosquera, D., & Steele, K. (2017). Complex trauma, dissociation and Borderline Personality Disorder: Working with integration failures. *European Journal of Trauma & Dissociation, 1*(1), 63–71. https://doi.org/10.1016/j.ejtd.2017.01.010

Muthane, U. (2011). Predictive genetic testing in Huntington's disease. *Annals of Indian Academy of Neurology, 14*(Suppl 1), S29–S30. https://doi.org/10.4103/0972-2327.83098

Nanni, V., Uher, R., & Danese, A. (2012). Childhood maltreatment predicts unfavorable course of illness and treatment outcome in depression: A meta-analysis. *American Journal of Psychiatry, 169*(2), 141–151.

Neria, Y., Olfson, M., Gameroff, M. J., Wickramaratne, P., Pilowsky, D., Verdeli, H., … Weissman, M. M. (2008). Trauma exposure and posttraumatic stress disorder among primary care patients with bipolar spectrum disorder. *Bipolar Disorders, 10*(4), 503–510.

Okkels, N., Trabjerg, B., Arendt, M., & Pedersen, C. B. (2016). Traumatic stress disorders and risk of subsequent schizophrenia spectrum disorder or bipolar disorder: A nationwide cohort study. *Schizophrenia Bulletin, 43*(1), 180–186.

Palmier-Claus, J. E., Berry, K., Bucci, S., Mansell, W., & Varese, F. (2016). Relationship between childhood adversity and bipolar affective disorder; Systematic review and meta-analysis. *The British Journal of Psychiatry, 209*(6), 454–459.

Paulsen, J. S. (2010). Early detection of Huntington Disease. *Future Neurology, 5*(1). https://doi.org/10.2217/fnl.09.78

Pavon, G., & Vaes, J. (2017). Bio-genetic vs. psycho-environmental conceptions of schizophrenia and their role in perceiving patients in human terms. *Psychosis, 9*(3), 245–253.

Pearce, J., Simpson, J., Berry, K., Bucci, S., Moskowitz, A., & Varese, F. (2017). Attachment and dissociation as mediators of the link between childhood trauma and psychotic experiences. *Clinical Psychology & Psychotherapy, 24*(6), 1304–1312.

Perez, J., Russo, D. A., Stochl, J., Shelley, G. F., Crane, C. M., Painter, M., … Jones, P. B. (2016). Understanding causes of and developing effective interventions for schizophrenia and other psychoses. *Programme Grants for Applied Research, No. 4.2.* Retrieved from https://www.ncbi.nlm.nih.gov/books/NBK350254/. doi:https://doi.org/10.3310/pgfar04020

Phelan, J. C., Yang, L. H., & Cruz-Rojas, R. (2006). Effects of attributing serious mental illnesses to genetic causes on orientations to treatment. *Psychiatric Services, 57*(3), 382–387.

Pickersgill, M., Niewöhner, J., Müller, R., Martin, P., & Cunningham-Burley, S. (2013). Mapping the new molecular landscape: Social dimensions of epigenetics. *New Genetics and Society, 32*(4), 429–447. https://doi.org/10.1080/14636778.2013.861739

Pies, R. W. (2011, July). Psychiatry's new brain-mind and the legend of the "chemical imbalance". *Psychiatric Times.* Retrieved from http://www.psychiatrictimes.com/blogs/psychiatry-new-brain-mind-and-legend-chemical-imbalance

Poulin, M. J., & Holman, E. A. (2013). Helping hands, healthy body? Oxytocin receptor gene and prosocial behavior interact to buffer the association between stress and physical health. *Hormones and Behavior, 63*(3), 510–517 https://doi.org/10.1016/j.yhbeh.2013.01.004

Powers, A., Fani, N., Cross, D., Ressler, K. J., & Bradley, B. (2016). Childhood trauma, PTSD, and psychosis: Findings from a highly traumatized, minority sample. *Child Abuse & Neglect, 58*, 111–118.

Prasad, S., Bhatia, T., Kukshal, P., Nimgaonkar, V. L., Deshpande, S. N., & Thelma, B. K. (2017). Attempts to replicate genetic associations with schizophrenia in a cohort from north India. *NPJ Schizophrenia, 3*, 28. https://doi.org/10.1038/s41537-017-0030-8

Prata, D., Mechelli, A., & Kapur, S. (2014). Clinically meaningful biomarkers for psychosis: A systematic and quantitative review. *Neuroscience and Biobehavioral Reviews, 45*, 134–141.

Read, J. (2010). Can poverty drive you mad? 'Schizophrenia', socio-economic status and the case for primary prevention. *New Zealand Journal of Psychology, 39*(2), 7–19.

Read, J., Agar, K., Argyle, N., & Aderhold, V. (2003). Sexual and physical abuse during childhood and adulthood as predictors of hallucinations, delusions and thought disorder. *Psychology and Psychotherapy: Theory, Research and Practice, 76*(1), 1–22.

Read, J., Fosse, R., Moskowitz, A., & Perry, B. (2014). The traumagenic neuro-developmental model of psychosis revisited. *Neuropsychiatry, 4*(1), 65–79.

Read, J., van Os, J., Morrison, A. P., & Ross, C. A. (2005). Childhood trauma, psychosis, and schizophrenia: A literature review with theoretical and clinical implications. *Acta Psychiatrica Scandinavica, 112*, 330–350.

Richardson, K. (2017). GWAS and cognitive abilities: Why correlations are inevitable and meaningless. *EMBO Reports.* https://doi.org/10.15252/embr.201744140

Richardson, L., Hameed, Y., Perez, J., Jones, P. B., & Kirkbride, J. B. (2017). Association of environment with the risk of developing psychotic disorders in rural populations: Findings from the social epidemiology of psychoses in East Anglia Study. *JAMA Psychiatry.* https://doi.org/10.1001/jamapsychiatry.2017.3582

Roberts, S., Keers, R., Lester, K. J., Coleman, J. R., Breen, G., Arendt, K., … Wong, C. C. (2015). HPA Axis related genes and response to psychological therapies: Genetics and epigenetics. *Depression and Anxiety, 32*(12), 861–870. https://doi.org/10.1002/da.22430

Roberts, S., Lester, K. J., Hudson, J. L., Rapee, R. M., Creswell, C., Cooper, P. J., … Eley, T. C. (2014). Serotonin transporter [corrected] methylation and response to cognitive behaviour therapy in children with anxiety disorders. *Translational Psychiatry, 16*(4), e444.

Ross, C. A., & Pam, A. (1995). *Pseudoscience in biological psychiatry.* New York, NY: John Wiley & Sons, Inc.

Rubanovich, A. V., & Khromov-Borisov, N. N. (2016). Genetic risk assessment of the joint effect of several genes: Critical appraisal. *Russian Journal of Genetics, 52*(7), 757–769.

Sawa, A., & Sedlak, T. W. (2016). Oxidative stress and inflammation in schizophrenia. *Schizophrenia Research, 176*, 1–2.

Sekar, A., Bialas, A. R., de Rivera, H., Davis, A., Hammond, T. R., Kamitaki, N., … McCarroll, S. A. (2016). Schizophrenia risk from complex variation of complement component 4. *Nature, 530*, 177. doi: https://doi.org/10.1038/nature16549 https://www.nature.com/articles/nature16549#supplementary-information

Selten, J. P., Booij, J., Buwalda, B., & Meyer-Lindenberg, A. (2017). Biological mechanisms whereby social exclusion may contribute to the etiology of psychosis: A narrative review. *Schizophrenia Bulletin, 43*(2), 276–292.

Shabalin, A. A., Anderson, J. S., Shade, J., Bakian, A., Darlington, T., Adkins, D. E., … Docherty, A. (2017). Genome-wide association study of suicide death: Results from the first wave of Utah completed suicide data. *bioRxiv.* https://doi.org/10.1101/234674

Shamseddeen, W., Asarnow, J. R., Clarke, G., Vitiello, B., Wagner, K. D., Birmaher, B., … Brent, D. A. (2011). Impact of physical and sexual abuse on treatment response in the treatment of resistant depression in adolescent study (TORDIA). *Journal of the American Academy of Child and Adolescent Psychiatry, 50*(3), 293–301. https://doi.org/10.1016/j.jaac.2010.11.019

Shevlin, M., Murphy, J., Read, J., Mallett, J., Adamson, G., & Houston, J. E. (2011). Childhood adversity and hallucinations: A community-based study using the National Comorbidity Survey Replication. *Social Psychiatry and Psychiatric Epidemiology, 46*(12), 1203–1210. https://doi.org/10.1007/s00127-010-0296-x

Singham, T., Viding, E., Schoeler, T., Arseneault, L., Ronald, A., Cecil, C. M., … Pingault, J. (2017). Concurrent and longitudinal contribution of exposure to bullying in childhood to mental health: The role of vulnerability and resilience. *JAMA Psychiatry, 74*(11), 1112–1119. https://doi.org/10.1001/jamapsychiatry.2017.2678

Snyder-Mackler, N., Sanz, J., Kohn, J. N., Brinkworth, J. F., Morrow, S., Shaver, A. O., … Tung, J. (2016). Social status alters immune regulation and response to infection in macaques. *Science, 354*(6315), 1041–1045.

Sprooten, E., Rasgon, A., Goodman, M., Carlin, A., Leibu, E., Lee, W. H., & Frangou, S. (2017). Addressing reverse inference in psychiatric neuroimaging: Meta-analyses of task-related brain activation in common mental disorders. *Human Brain Mapping, 38*(4), 1846–1864. https://doi.org/10.1002/hbm.23486

Stelmach, A., & Nerlich, B. (2015). Metaphors in search of a target: The curious case of epigenetics. *New Genetics and Society, 34*(2), 196–218. https://doi.org/10.1080/14636778.2015.1034849

Stern, D. B. (1996). Dissociation and constructivism: Commentary on papers by Davies and Harris. *Psychoanalytic Dialogues, 6*(2), 251–266.

Sugaya, L., Hasin, D. S., Olfson, M., Lin, K. H., Grant, B. F., & Blanco, C. (2012). Child physical abuse and adult mental health: A national study. *Journal of Traumatic Stress, 25*(4), 384–392.

Sullivan, P. F., Kendler, K. S., & Neale, M. C. (2003). Schizophrenia as a complex trait: Evidence from a meta-analysis of twin studies. *Archives of General Psychiatry, 60*(12), 1187–1192. https://doi.org/10.1001/archpsyc.60.12.1187

Summerfield, D. A. (2017). Western depression is not a universal condition. *The British Journal of Psychiatry, 211*(1), 52–52. https://doi.org/10.1192/bjp.211.1.52

Teicher, M. H., Anderson, C. M., & Polcari, A. (2012). Childhood maltreatment is associated with reduced volume in the hippocampal subfields CA3, dentate gyrus, and subiculum. *Proceedings of the National Academy of Sciences, 109*(9), E563–E572. https://doi.org/10.1073/pnas.1115396109

Teicher, M. H., & Samson, J. A. (2013). Childhood maltreatment and psychopathology: A case for ecophenotypic variants as clinically and neurobiologically distinct subtypes. *The American Journal of Psychiatry, 170*(10), 1114–1133.

Teicher, M. H., & Samson, J. A. (2016). Annual research review: Enduring neurobiological effects of childhood abuse and neglect. *Journal of Child Psychology and Psychiatry, 57*(3), 241–266.

van Dam, D. S., van Nierop, M., Viechtbauer, W., Velthorst, E., van Winkel, R., Genetic Risk Outcome of Psychosis (GROUP) investigators, … Wiersma, D. (2015). Childhood abuse and neglect in relation to the presence and persistence of psychotic and depressive symptomatology. *Psychological Medicine, 45*(7), 1363–1377. https://doi.org/10.1017/s0033291714001561

van der Kolk, B. A., Brown, P., & van der Hart, O. (1989). Pierre Janet on posttraumatic stress. *Journal of Traumatic Stress, 2*(4), 365–378.

van Winkel, R., van Nierop, M., Myin-Germeys, I., & van Os, J. (2012). Childhood trauma as a cause of psychosis: Linking genes, psychology and biology. *Canadian Journal of Psychiatry, 58*(1), 44–51.

Varese, F., Smeets, F., Drukker, M., Lieverse, R., Lataster, T., Viechtbauer, W., … Bentall, R. P. (2012). Childhood adversities increase the risk of psychosis: A meta-analysis of patient-control, prospective- and cross-sectional cohort studies. *Schizophrenia Bulletin, 38*(4), 661–671. https://doi.org/10.1093/schbul/sbs050

Vassos, E., Di Forti, M., Coleman, J., Iyegbe, C., Prata, D., Euesden, J., … Breen, G. (2017). An examination of polygenic score risk prediction in individuals with first-episode psychosis. *Biological Psychiatry, 81*(6), 470–477. https://doi.org/10.1016/j.biopsych.2016.06.028

Venkatasubramanian, G., & Keshavan, M. S. (2016). Biomarkers in psychiatry – A critique. *Annals of Neurosciences, 23*(1), 3–5.

Wallace, S., Nazroo, J., & Becares, L. (2016). Cumulative effect of racial discrimination on the mental health of ethnic minorities in the United Kingdom. *American Journal of Public Health, 106*(7), 1294–1300.

Whitaker, R. (2010). *Anatomy of an epidemic: Magic bullets, psychiatric drugs and the astonishing rise of mental illness.* New York: Broadway Paperbacks.

Willhite, R. K., Niendam, T. A., Bearden, C. E., Zinberg, J., O'Brien, M. P., & Cannon, T. D. (2008). Gender differences in symptoms, functioning and social support in patients at ultra-high risk for developing a psychotic disorder. *Schizophrenia Research, 104,* 237–245.

Zhang, X. Y., Chen, D. C., Xiu, M. H., Yang, F. D., Haile, C. N., Kosten, T. A., & Kosten, R. R. (2012). Gender differences in never-medicated first-episode schizophrenia and medicated chronic schizophrenia patients. *Journal of Clinical Psychiatry, 73*(7), 1025–1033.

PART II

The Clinical Experience

Theoretical arguments about biology, trauma, terminology, and the meaning of life and suffering are all well and good, but when it comes to the practical issues of *what to do*, clinicians, family members, and individuals seeking help just want answers and direction. Of course, the most difficult idea to swallow sometimes is that there is no concrete, certain solution for most people; what helps one person harms another, and the process of understanding and knowing what might be helpful for any given individual is usually a long one with many veering detours along the way. Often, what helps people through their suffering, distress, and angst is not some technical intervention or invention but rather human relationship, exercise and nutrition, insight and wisdom, compassion, and learning to love oneself. This second part explores what some people tend to find helpful, barriers to getting this help, and how this may or may not sync with professional ideas of what is helpful and/or necessary. It also covers what most definitely is NOT helpful, and ways in which the system can do better. Hopefully, these chapters can provide some direction and resources to guide individuals and clinicians towards a healing and non-destructive path.

CHAPTER 7

Finding Help

> I went through about seven or eight therapists because you can't, I couldn't find one that really helped. P4
>
> Accessing treatment services ... can be a bloody nightmare. P5

Some of the standard psychotherapeutic approaches experienced by individuals who have suffered developmental and other trauma include dialectical behavior therapy (DBT); cognitive behavioral therapy (CBT); trauma-informed psychodynamic and relational therapies; phase-based, trauma-specific therapy approaches; DID-specific therapy; cognitive behavior therapy for psychosis (CBT-p); Internal Family Systems (IFS); and adjunctive therapies, such as art therapy, modified eye movement desensitization and reprocessing (EMDR), somatic therapies, and hypnosis. Each of these treatment approaches has demonstrated or has a theoretical history of effectiveness for particular phenomena. Though, at the same time, critics of opposing specialty areas tend to accuse many of these various brands of being oversold, methodologically flawed, and any statistical significance in outcomes as representing a small minority of those seeking help (e.g., McKenna & Kingdon, 2014; Shedler, 2015). This is despite the evidence demonstrating that most standard practices are about as effective as any other (Hawton et al., 2016; Steinert, Munder, Rabung, Hoyer, & Falk, 2017). Further, most outcome and review studies tend to find differences in effectiveness along the lines of ideological allegiance as opposed to there being evidence of objective superiority or inferiority of particular approaches (Fonagy, 2015; Leichsenring & Steinert, 2017).

© The Author(s) 2018
N. Hunter, *Trauma and Madness in Mental Health Services*,
https://doi.org/10.1007/978-3-319-91752-8_7

Many consumer advocates and ex-patients, as well as most of the participants, have asserted that these approaches can, at times, be experienced as
rigid, invalidating, and lacking meaning or may be helpful or harmful at
different times in the work (e.g., Swift, Tompkins, & Parkin, 2017).
Additionally, the effectiveness of both psychotherapy and pharmaceutical
interventions are largely reliant on placebo/nocebo effects and the therapeutic relationship, independent of technique or presenting issues (Ardito
& Rabellino, 2011; Faria et al., 2017; Zilcha-Mano, Roose, Barber, &
Rutherford, 2015). In other words, what one thinks about the power of the
intervention, rather than the intervention itself, often determines how effective that intervention is. Repeatedly, service users describe finding help in
spite of, rather than because of, standard mental health services, and plead
for trauma-informed collaborative, relationship-focused, client-directed,
non-medical approaches that honor the subjective experience and frame
atypical experiences as adaptive coping tools for an overwhelming and most
often traumatic environment (Cohen, 2005; McEnteggart, Barnes-Holmes,
Dillon, Egger, & Oliver, 2017; McHugh, Whitton, Peckham, Welge, &
Otto, 2013; Mead & Copeland, 2000; Mehl-Madrona, Jul, & Mainguy,
2014; Williams, 2012; Williamson, 2009). At the same time, it is rare that
such services are encountered; in fact, it most often is quite the opposite.

COMMON EXPERIENCES WITHIN THE SYSTEM

It's been that awful … the mental health services have probably been as
much if not more of a threat to recovery and feeling ok with myself than all
of my traumas have been. And they've certainly been highly traumatic. P5
　　There was a few times where I went into the emergency department
because I was really dissociated, and sort of forgot where I lived and who I
was … a lot of them didn't take me seriously … so I didn't get any treatment
for a while because I wasn't being taken seriously. P8
　　I joke and tell people that I keep going back in [to the hospital] so I can
see how much they've advanced. Which, I hate to say, they haven't advanced
very much on a lot of things. P10
　　There were so many mistakes made along the way … it was traumatic. It
was re-traumatizing … there was just mistake after mistake after mistake
made. P12

A common experience for people navigating the mental health system
is finding that they spend many years, sometimes decades, working with
numerous mental health and general health practitioners who often are

unable to help them and/or do not take them seriously (e.g., National Health Service, 2015). In addition, clinicians will often refuse to work with particular individuals, especially if they carry certain diagnoses, such as schizophrenia, BPD, or DID. This is actually considered ethical practice—clinicians may refuse treatment based on a lack of "competency" and choose to not work with someone who carries a particular diagnosis. It is surely important that clinicians feel competent to work with the people who come to them for help and they certainly have the right to assert their boundaries as to particular individuals with whom they may not feel comfortable working. But, based on the lack of validity and discriminatory nature of diagnoses, doing so based on a label is a serious problem. Further, why are so many clinicians incompetent to work with those who tend to be in the greatest need of help?

To be told that one is too difficult, treatment-resistant, or noncompliant and, in turn, having services refused can be detrimental. Two participants, both diagnosed with psychotic disorders, spoke of trying to get couples therapy that instead resulted in "right from the beginning [being] told ... that there was no way that they could help me and that I was too complicated or too complex of a situation" (P3) and "the guy wouldn't talk to me ... because I wasn't on my medication" (P10). This can leave a person feeling rejected, hopeless, defective, and re-traumatized. Indeed, many people who encounter the mental health system find that the experience can be even worse than the original trauma and suffering for which they were seeking help.

Sometimes, the patient must teach the doctor how to work with dissociated parts, self-harm, substance use, strange belief systems, or any other phenomena that a professional has difficulty understanding and has never been trained to work with beyond suppressing it with a pill. This may be frustrating for some service users; for others this can actually be a rewarding experience when the clinician is willing to collaborate and learn from those he or she is working with. While it can be helpful for a clinician to be open to new experiences and to learning, more often service users tend to be confronted with clinicians who are authoritarian, coercive, and/or perhaps too adherent to preexisting frameworks and theoretical ideas to the point of seeing what they want to see rather than what is truly before them.

Individuals who experience intense emotional distress and/or atypical experiences tend to also have more frequent contact with intrusive, coercive, and restrictive forms of intervention. Interestingly, these same interventions are associated with increased suicide, with the greater association with restrictive care being associated with the greatest risk of suicide (Hjorthoj, Madsen, Agerbo, & Nordentoft, 2014). Turns out that visitations to the psychiatric emergency room are directly related to an *increased* likelihood of future suicidality, independent of severity of distress or initial presentation (Coyle, Shaver, & Linehan, 2018). One possibility for this association is the common experience of service users feeling invalidated, stigmatized and othered, dismissed, and/or misunderstood because of preexisting frameworks, judgments, and assumptions made by mental health professionals.

Additionally, many may find that because they appear calm and functional, their internal distress must not be as severe as expressed, or that there is an assumption that a person is "fine" if they happened to appear well in the therapy session. As one participant stated, "I'm actually on disability and a lot of people don't get that because I don't look sick. So, they're confused by it and think I'm just scamming the system or something" (P3). In fact, it is common for individuals who are not obviously dysfunctional or acutely psychotic to be invalidated, dismissed, or accused of attention-seeking when they express their intense pain and suffering and seek help. At the same time, trauma and dissociative disorder specialists have recognized this problem, for *some*, and have developed important guidelines and interventions that promote greater awareness of the effects of trauma and challenge the status quo within services throughout all levels of care. The need for trauma-informed practices in all areas of medicine is an almost universally recommended need by service users and conscientious clinicians alike.

PROFESSIONAL RECOMMENDATIONS AND GUIDELINES

Hold frameworks lightly, and accept the notion that they aren't truth but models of what we think the truth is and that they can co-exist and they can overlap and they can also be different and that's ok. P5

There is a huge association with having someone give you a structure, having to function within that ... I sort of take a very ... submissive approach. P8

I mean I guess it would help if more mental health professionals were aware of dissociation ... because most of them aren't. And, I don't mind explaining and trying to help them understand, but a lot of them also just don't care. I think in the public system that's more of an issue. Well, I think they care on a service level, but they don't necessarily care enough to find out information, find out how to help or take the time to ask how they can help. P11

Standard practices within the mental health system dictate that the initial steps in working with individuals in distress are to evaluate symptoms, make a diagnosis, and create an appropriate treatment plan based on this diagnosis. There are specific guild guidelines within the various mental health specialties for most of the major *DSM* categories, such as schizophrenia, BPD, DID, PTSD, depression, and bipolar disorders. With this, there is the illusion of predictability, scientific certainty, and concrete steps toward improved well-being. Of course, as discussed at length in Chap. 4, such validity based on diagnoses does not exist. Nonetheless, the status quo remains.

The trauma and dissociative disorder fields have made great advances in providing guidelines that consider the complexity of the trauma response, the long-term, eclectic approach necessary for working with chronic or complex trauma, and the tremendous healing value of the therapeutic relationship. At the same time, those individuals who are not fortunate enough to be recognized as suffering the results of trauma or adversity, or if their presentation is un-understandable to the clinician, are likely to be recommended for intrusive and coercive interventions that tend to pathologize, invalidate, and stigmatize one's unique form of coping with and processing life. Naturally, there are some reductionistic and mechanistic approaches within the trauma field too (i.e., Prolonged Exposure Therapy), but this is not the norm for trauma-based approaches more generally. Overall, the recommendations and interventions designed for complex trauma have much to teach the broader mental health field and offer many useful insights and tools for working with traumatized populations.

Guidelines for Complex Trauma

The International Society for Traumatic Stress Studies offers a free consensus guide and comprehensive review of the empirical literature that was developed by professionals considered to be experts in complex trauma (Cloitre et al., 2012). The International Society for the Study of Trauma and Dissociation similarly has developed a set of guidelines specific to the diagnosis of DID that recommends a phase-based, individualized, eclectic approach based in psychodynamic relational principles (International

Society for the Study of Trauma and Dissociation, 2011). It is generally agreed upon, in this small specialty area, that a relational, flexible, long-term approach is necessary, and that particular components and techniques from CBT, as well as other adjunctive methods, are useful as tools within a psychodynamic framework (Howell, 2011; Steele, van der Hart, & Nijenhuis, 2001; van der Hart, Nijenhuis, & Steele, 2006). The recommendation for a psychodynamic framework is largely due to a typical adverse reaction to standard CBT approaches, such as exposure and/or short-term manualized treatment, by individuals who have experienced complex trauma and chronic adversity (Brand, Lanius, Vermetten, Loewenstein, & Spiegel, 2012), and the necessity of a secure attachment relationship for healing childhood trauma (Steele et al., 2001).

Treatments for DID and other complex trauma disorders are associated with decreases in dissociation, depression, PTSD, overall distress, drug use, physical pain, suicidality (Brand, Classen, Lanius, et al., 2009; Brand, Classen, McNary, & Zaveri, 2009), and Schneiderian first-rank symptoms (Ellason & Ross, 1997), with an average of 5–6 years in treatment (Coons & Bowman, 2001). Mosquera and Ross (2017) have suggested that implementing psychotherapy for the treatment of Schneiderian symptoms does not require differentiating whether such phenomena are purportedly "psychotic" versus "dissociative".

The limited number of studies, case reports, and qualitative studies that have focused on outcomes of these approaches have been criticized for being marred by bias (Piper & Merskey, 2005), lacking external and internal validity, being based on small sample sizes, and having extremely high attrition (Brand et al., 2012). Although there have been no randomized controlled studies looking at recovery and treatment with DID or complex trauma, it appears from much of the literature that only about 30% of people are significantly helped by these treatments, and many relapse within several years (Kluft, 2001; Myrick, Brand, & Putnam, 2013). Moreover, many individuals become significantly worse over the course of treatment (Myrick et al., 2013). This is not uncommon, however, as "evidence-based treatments" across diagnostic boundaries have approximately the same rates of improvement and regression (Shedler, 2015).

The guidelines demonstrate an understanding for the importance of working with, instead of trying to get rid of, one's unique way of understanding the world and the self. The overt presentation or "symptoms" are not the primary focus; rather, the focus is on the cognitive, emotional, and psychodynamic characteristics, conflicts, and symbolizations that are represented by these "symptoms", including the dissociated personality states, for instance. Direct work with dissociated parts of the self is secondary to assisting the person to learn how to recognize, accept, and negotiate directly with these aspects of his or her self on one's own (van der Hart et al., 2006). Often, the client is aided in understanding his or her overall internal self rather than discrete personality parts. Nonetheless, working with parts in order to maintain safety, control maladaptive behaviors, and understand the individual's past and present interpersonal relationships and memories at times becomes an essential focus. It is recognized that working directly with one's presenting issues, such as "alters", is necessary even if it may temporarily increase dissociation and/or dysfunction (Harper, 2011).

These guidelines suggest a specific three-phased approach consisting of: (1) an initial focus on psychoeducation, coping skills, safety, and identification of and stabilization of unsafe behaviors and/or suicidal tendencies, whether the individual is amnestic for such behaviors or not; (2) a focus on working through traumatic material in a gradual, non-linear manner that acknowledges the periodic need to return to phase 1 issues and the need to include all parts of the individual's identity; and finally, (3) integration of the psyche, skill and relationship building, and a focus on psychosocial issues and everyday life. It is highly recommended that stabilization of "symptoms" and development of the therapeutic relationship need to be established before memories can be addressed or worked on directly. It is also important that throughout each phase, the therapist constantly aide the person in staying aware in the present. These phases are not thought to be linear, nor are they mutually exclusive.

Most treatments that are specific to the DID diagnosis or other complex trauma disorders focus on resolving traumatic cognitions and emotion dysregulation, enhancing harmony between dissociated personality states, and achieving integration of all dissociated parts and memories of the individual (Cloitre et al., 2012; Courtois, 2004; Gleaves, 1996; International Society for the Study of Trauma and Dissociation, 2011). However, integration of subjectively separate parts of the self is not always obtained or the goal of treatment, and co-consciousness, or internal communication and harmony, may be more important (Hegeman, 2009). The idea of integration is particularly complex when viewed from the perspective that all individuals have multiple self-states (e.g., Kurzban, 2010).

It also is understood that individuals frequently deny or have persistent doubts about the truth of memories and subjective experiences, especially when it is in regard to parental figures (Davies, 1996; Freyd, 1994; Howell, 2011). What appears to be imperative is that the clinician enter the relationship with complete authenticity and tolerance for withstanding the stories of the horrors and injustices that led to contradictory and confusing behaviors, which can far exceed that which may occur with clients presenting with less severe distress or dysfunction (e.g., Hegeman, 2009; Steele, van der Hart, & Nijenhuis, 2005). Further, clinicians must be able to tolerate uncertainty and not insist upon the factual correctness of confusing memories or experiences.

As with everything in the mental health field, though, there exists a political battle across orientations as to specific terminology, techniques, and what "must" be done for recovery to occur (Hegeman, 2009). Further, what constitutes "recovery" is highly subjective and means greatly different things across specialties and among professionals versus individuals with lived experience (Dinniss, Roberts, Hubbard, Hounsell, & Webb, 2007; Neil et al., 2009; Shumway et al., 2003). Generally, these guidelines tend to be, perhaps, overly structured and leave little room for allowing the client to lead the process or consider some individualized needs, such as not ever directly exposing oneself to the original trauma. There is a strong insistence on the importance of making traumatic memories conscious (e.g., van der Hart et al., 2006) and focusing on repetitive discussion of traumatic experiences, despite the increased chances of re-traumatization and becoming trapped in the past (e.g., van der Kolk, 1989, 2014).

However, these guidelines and frameworks provide many useful suggestions that can be generalized across *DSM* categories, even if they rarely are. Similarly, psychoanalytic treatments designed for "schizophrenia" have also been suggested by many clinicians to be generalizable across more severe or intense experiences not generally considered to be "neurotic" (Gainer, 1994; Karon, 2003; Kirshner, 2015; Silver, 2003; Sinason & Silver, 2008). Further, many individuals who were once considered "borderline schizophrenic" also have a long history of treatment within a psychoanalytic framework, suggesting the universal possibilities of these approaches and the need for more collaboration across specialties (Baker & Baker, 1987; Connor, Nelson, Walterfang, Velakoulis, & Thompson, 2009; Kernberg, 1976; Kohut, 1977; Tuttman, 1990).

Psychodynamic aspects of treatment tend to focus on identifying enactments (or patterns of unconscious interpersonal interactions and behaviors) and interpreting them as indicative of a person's internal world and past experiences (Bromberg, 1998; Davies & Frawley, 1991; Stern, 2004). The approach emphasizes increasing internal strength and encouraging age-appropriate behavior while validating traumatic experiences and associated confusion and pain. Additionally, the attachment relationship and the events that occur between the therapist and client are central to the treatment (Bromberg, 1995; Davies, 1996; Hegeman, 2009; Howell, 2011; Stern, 2004).

Attunement to non-verbal communication and encouragement of more presently adaptive coping strategies is also a fundamental part of both psychodynamic and cognitive approaches, as well as psychiatry, on the whole (Foley & Gentile, 2010; Steele et al., 2005). Addressing cognitive distortions and physiological hyperarousal are also universal treatment goals across diagnoses and orientations (Cloitre et al., 2012; Harper, 2011; Morrison, 2001; Steele et al., 2005). The overt phenomena, whether it be confusing behaviors, distorted beliefs, voices, dissociated parts of self, excessive energy or anxiety, obsessions, and so on., can all be seen as providing some function (i.e., to express otherwise unacceptable emotions or experiences, to confuse and distance, to cope with overwhelming anxiety, etc.) and need not divert the overall focus on enactments, emotional reactions on the part of the therapist, symbolic and thematic patterns that may represent unconscious or dissociated emotions and experiences, and internal conflicts. In general, trauma-informed approaches that focus on recovery, empowerment, meaning-making, and reducing distress, rather than on "symptoms", appear to be effective for many in decreasing overt distress or atypical beliefs/behaviors, suicidality, and increasing functioning (Bacon & Kennedy, 2015; Farkas, 2007; Morrison, 2009; Ross & Keyes, 2004; Varese, Udachina, Myin-Germeys, Oorschot, & Bentall, 2011).

Adjunctive techniques, such as meditation, relaxation exercises, or EMDR, as well as standard CBT or DBT skills-based exercises, such as documenting patterns and triggers, exposure to anxiety-inducing experiences, and challenging automatic thoughts, can be incorporated throughout depending on the specific dominating psychic phenomena, but need not be the sole focus or override the deeper work of focusing on how these behaviors or atypical experiences represent internal pain and conflict (e.g., Mosquera & Ross, 2017). The overt phenomena must be acknowledged and understood, not suppressed and pathologized, no matter what the specific phenomena may be.

The Power Threat Meaning Framework

The Division of Clinical Psychology of the British Psychological Society has recently released a comprehensive framework for working with individuals in distress that is trauma-informed, and attempts to provide an alternative to diagnoses and medical conceptualizations of emotional distress and atypical experiences (Johnstone et al., 2018). While it is not necessarily a formal intervention or guideline, it nonetheless is a broad framework that can inform professional services across specialties. This revolutionary publication not only considers overt trauma, such as child abuse, it also incorporates evidence about the role of power and oppression, social adversity, and the utility of meaning-making and personal narratives. In general, it seeks to make central the link between emotional distress and social injustice, while focusing on helping people make meaning of their experiences, challenging the greater societal status quo, and valuing the adaptive nature of atypical experiences, such as hearing voices, and diversity of personality and coping. It offers an approach to identifying patterns in distress that is not diagnostically based, and applies to all of us at times, not just a specific group designated as "mentally ill".

By appreciating the adaptive and understandable nature of one's emotional and behavioral reactions to adversity and injustice, it allows for interventions focused on building on the individual's strengths, hearing and validating one's narrative story, helping to create hope and foster societal change, decreasing shame and hopelessness, increasing self-worth and compassion, and building relationship and community. In this broad framework, individual preferences for what "works" is honored and includes various forms of psychotherapy, psychiatric drugs, peer support, art, music, yoga, nutrition, exercise, activism, and more. Mental health professionals are seen as having a helpful, but not necessary or all-important, role in working through one's past and creating meaning and new ways of coping. It also honors creative and non-Western cultural perspectives. Perhaps most profound, and relevant to the discourse outlined throughout this book, is that this framework was developed in an egalitarian collaboration with trauma and psychiatric survivors rather than being explicitly "expert" driven.

In addition to this broad overarching framework, the British Psychological Society has also put out a set of guidelines on the use of language and supports the use of alternatives to medicalized diagnoses (The British Psychological Society, 2014). Lucy Johnstone (2014, 2017) and colleagues in the United Kingdom advocate for the use of psychological case conceptualizations that honor the individual and take into account unique strengths and problem areas instead of pathologizing and reductionistic illness language that lacks meaning and often leads to stigma and hopelessness. They suggest relying on an evolving, collaborative psychosocial formulation of an individual's distinctive constellation of difficulties in the context of their life experiences and within the client's frame of reference and meaning. This is a client-led process that validates subjective experience, is flexible, and is constantly adapting to the person's changing needs. A psychological formulation does not make assumptions, is collaborative, is flexible and evolving throughout treatment, and includes strengths and weaknesses of an individual's behaviors and responses to their past and current life.

How Clinicians Can Make a Difference

I've found that it's been very helpful when therapists don't act like they're the authority figure and they're calling all the shots. P1

Of course, the relationship is what is the healing part, 'cause you can't trust people very easily when they have been so challenging to deal with. I can't. P4

It's not really so much what I'd want them to know, it's who I want them to be ... If they're a human being, and they're in touch with that, and they're willing to connect with me, we can work and we can do good stuff. That's not to say that specific knowledge can't be brilliant ... but, it's really who they are and not so much what they know that's the key thing for me. P5

It goes back to flexibility—you can't generalize really anything. It's all about what's right in the moment or what's right for you, specifically, and what's right one time might be wrong another time. P8

For every individual, the goals are going to be somewhat different. P12

Any given individual is going to be helped by a different combination of interventions and therapeutic features. People are complex, and so the various ways in which one might heal or recover, as well as the numerous factors that contribute to any given individual's unique constellation of difficulties, are also complex. Any therapeutic intervention, therefore, must be individualized, flexible, and focused on attunement and a healthy therapeutic relationship. Throughout the course of the therapeutic process, it may be imperative to collaborate with the client and honor his or her own subjective experience while also holding lightly one's own framework or perspectives.

A client-directed, humanistic, collaborative framework for working with distressed individuals has been advocated for by many service users and professionals across all fields of psychiatric and psychological study (Cohen, 2005; Duncan, Miller, & Sparks, 2004; Gibson, Brand, Burt, Boden, & Benson, 2013). The importance of having a framework that honors the subjective experience of the individual and does not force one to frame things or behave in a way that the mental health professional would prefer cannot be underestimated. There can be immeasurable meaning and healing potential in being recognized and acknowledged for the individual and unique person that one is, rather than being forced or encouraged to be that which someone else assumes or wishes one to be (Rogers, 1961/1995; Winnicott, 1965/1990).

In general, there is no one "right" way to work with people, and even the "right" way may not be the right way all of the time. Considering the political battles within the mental health field, this message is an important one to convey. Even the methods and interventions that appear to be agreed upon within the field as absolutely necessary for recovery may not be so absolute. For instance, it is taken for granted that a phased-based protocol, which includes specific work on trauma memories and delays a central focus on everyday problems and building relationships to the final phase, is the best treatment course for individuals who are recovering from complex trauma. First-person perspectives, however, do not necessarily support such a supposition.

For many, working on stabilization and skill building, while simultaneously building trust in the therapeutic relationship is, indeed, an important first phase of treatment, as it is for any person presenting for therapy. After that, however, it becomes very individualized. Many participants found it countertherapeutic to dwell on the traumatic past at the expense of focusing on current experiences and understanding how the past relates to the present. For some, learning to live in the present, making meaning, finding purpose, developing healthy relationships, and engaging in rewarding activities were principal factors in the healing process, often above and beyond those typically attended to in "trauma therapy".

Focused discussion on trauma memories or pushing to remember events that are hazy or even forgotten is not an imperative for successful treatment. Pushing for or focusing on memories is not always necessary or even helpful, although it is important that there be space for memories to be discussed if and when the person decides it is time to discuss them. A gentle balance of pushing versus not pushing is important, though, as avoidance is a common coping mechanism for most; however, this is very individualized and should be based on attunement and collaboration rather than an authoritarian or protocol-driven insistence upon such (e.g., Bjornestad et al., 2017). There is a difference between supporting a person to acknowledge and deal with what is there and pushing and digging for what is not or forcing a person to relive or see things that are better left unseen.

This is a particularly significant point, considering that there is currently little dispute that memories are fallible (e.g., Koriat, Goldsmith, & Pansky, 2000), certain practices (such as hypnosis) can lead to distorted memories (e.g., Scoboria, Mazzoni, Kirsch, & Milling, 2002), emotional memories may be consciously experienced through symbolic metaphor (e.g., Modell, 2005), and that it is essential that professionals refrain from endorsing the literal truth or lack thereof of early memories because of these issues (APA Working Group on Investigation of Memories of Childhood Abuse, 1998).

It is important for individuals to feel validated, but also that they learn to trust their own sense of reality without a professional suggesting what may or may not have happened. The goal for many is to learn to trust the self, to learn to tolerate not knowing, and to acknowledge and accept their emotions as meaningful reactions to life events without needing to "recover memories" or be certain in order to do so. Recommendations by some specialists to bring traumatic memories into consciousness (van der Hart et al., 2006), guide graduated exposure to memories (Steele & van der Hart, 2009), or help with doubts regarding the truth of memories through literal interpretations of transference-countertransference reactions and work with dissociated parts (e.g., Howell, 2011) need to be considered with caution, particularly bearing in mind that few find this to be an explicit goal or even helpful in their overall healing process. What appears most helpful is focusing on emotions and learning to have compassion for self-parts in the context in which their experiences developed, however ambiguous this context may be.

Clinicians need to be able to tolerate ambiguity and uncertainty while still maintaining a supportive and validating demeanor. Clinicians should avoid telling a client what they have or have not experienced (memories, psychologically, or otherwise). This is especially true when considering the common tendency for abused individuals to do and say what they perceive is expected of them, as well as the common problem of clients generally lying to their therapist and telling them what they think they want to hear

(Blanchard & Farber, 2016). The power that authority has in shaping individuals' behaviors and beliefs is something that must be acknowledged and treated with care. Having a person believe in one's capabilities, an ability to recover, and in one's humanity and goodness is incredibly healing. Just as powerful, though, are the "nocebo" messages of disbelief, hopelessness, helplessness, dependency, and defectiveness that are so often given by mental health professionals (Greville-Harris & Dieppe, 2015).

In fact, beyond any other factors, the clinician's personal characteristics and the therapeutic relationship are key factors in determining whether treatment is helpful or harmful (e.g., Fluckiger, Del Re, Wampold, Symonds, & Horvath, 2012). Specifically, clients find it important for a therapist to be genuine, honest, and to foster trust and safety above all else. The relationship needs to be authentic, empowering, and respectful in order to promote growth and recovery. Attunement is also key. When a mental health professional is able to tolerate emotions, control his or her own reactions, and truly hear and see what the client is trying to express or need, then the client can begin to trust that the clinician will be there and be supportive when in need. Moreover, attunement may help the client to better understand and trust his or her self while also feeling deeply understood by a genuinely present and familiar other.

Additionally, it is important that the therapist cares for his or her own inner selves, demonstrates healthy emotional expression, and is honest about limits and boundaries. Being genuine and respectful is not the same thing as being passive or always *nice*. In fact, some participants found that setting limits explicitly allowed for the establishment of trust and motivation. The therapeutic relationship can serve as a model for how individuals could improve relationships with others. In addition to external relationships, it is important to facilitate healthy interactions with the self and with and between dissociated parts of the self; modeling can be a potent tool for this. Many people who have grown up experiencing developmental adversity had poor role models, and so being able to learn how to have a healthy range of emotional experiences without breaking down or judging oneself can be invaluable.

Collaboration and egalitarianism, as well as openness and authenticity on the part of the clinician, are central to effective implementation of psychotherapy (e.g., Galbusera & Kyselo, 2017) and are generally preferred by service users (e.g., Byrne & Morrison, 2014; Topor & Denhov, 2015). While the clinician's theoretical framework is helpful in guiding treatment, providing some direction, and helping to offer some meaning-making ideas, it is not objective fact and is specific to the clinician's own cultural and developmental experiences and worldviews. And so, being open to the ways in which individuals frame their own experiences or make sense of these experiences is imperative. A flexible, individualized framework for working with people in distress necessitates patience, openness, safety, trust, honesty, and shared connections. It further requires equality and mutuality, rather than a top-down, expert/patient dynamic, within a real relationship with a real person who is willing to hold a safe space and have the patience and understanding to not direct or push agendas or specific outcomes. This also allows for clients to learn how to want to help themselves and to discover what is authentic to their self versus trying to be what another person wants them to be.

Additionally, clinicians need to be willing to work within the defensive system any individual is presenting with, no matter how fantastical or bizarre it may seem to the outsider. Trying to change a person right away or force the person to take on the perspectives of the therapist denies the ways in which the person has come to survive within his or her world and only results in rigid clinging to these defenses. Working with a person's dissociated parts, or voices, especially considering that we all have such parts to different degrees of dissociation, is essential. In particular, hearing what these parts have to say, understanding what experiences they represent, and bringing to awareness the conflicts represented by them is an important part of the process, rather than trying to get rid of them (e.g., Bromberg, 1998). Even if a person is acutely paranoid or having implausible beliefs, such as the CIA has implanted chips in their brain for purposes of surveillance, this still can be honored and worked within in a safe manner. A clinician can help the person figure out ways to protect his or herself, such as collaborating on ideas of blocking the signals or understanding what it is that person believes he or she needs to hide in the first place. What are they afraid of the CIA finding out? In none of these methods does a clinician have to explicitly agree or disagree with the reality of the client. More than anything, building compassion for the self and self-parts of a person in distress is necessary for growth and recovery; shaming people for what they believe and how they behave does not build compassion.

It is understood that some mental health professionals might find it frightening to let go of authority or to allow themselves to be confused or uncertain without resolution, especially when they are being paid for their supposed expertise and help. For sure, the clinician also has his or her own defensive structure that prevents overwhelming existential anxiety to consume their being.[1] Further, clinicians are bound by constraints of the government and insurance companies. Yet, when working with individuals who have experienced chronic adversity, oppression, and/or trauma, it is essential that the professional can withstand the stories of helplessness, terror, and injustice without immediately trying to "fix" the situation, regardless of demands otherwise. Clinicians need to tolerate ambiguity, have genuine curiosity (rather than "expertise"), and serve as witnesses without "freaking out". Participant 4 could not begin to express how powerful it was for her to "just have a person in that space, that fearful, sad, angry space. Like a witnessing." Just simply being there can sometimes be enough.

It also is essential that clinicians be aware that a person's outer presentation often does not reflect his or her internal experience, and it also may not correspond with experiences between sessions. Additionally, people may have different needs in how they communicate, and this may not always be verbal. For example, some may prefer to use imagery, use art-based tools, to walk around while talking, or write out their thoughts instead of speaking. Journaling and sharing journal entries from throughout the week is another tool that individuals find helpful to give a fuller picture of one's day-to-day struggles.

Flexibility within the psychotherapeutic relationship and process also appears to be particularly vital. People who have experienced developmental adversity and oppression have an understandably difficult time tolerating rigidity and rules that do not consider their individual needs. Sometimes this might include having flexibility with the frame and boundaries of therapy, of course while still honoring the limits of the clinician, such as offering between-session contact, creative ways of conducting therapy (like taking a walk), occasional extension of time when needed, and, for some, even appropriate touching, like a hug. Flexibility also includes being attuned to the client's changing needs and finding the balance between pushing and supporting.

Creating and understanding meaning within a person's experience allows for a greater respect for the varieties of experience and also validates the real experiences underlying seemingly bizarre beliefs or behaviors (Boevink & Corstens, 2012; Geekie & Read, 2009; Randal et al., 2009). Increasingly, and largely outside of the United States, researchers are suggesting the need for treatments that focus on specific complaints (i.e., voices, paranoia, amnesia, depersonalization, depressed mood, manic states, and so on) rather than broader classifications or generalized protocols (e.g., Barch et al., 2013; Bentall, 2003; Johnstone, 2014). Additionally, trauma-informed interventions have been shown to be effectively and safely used within psychiatric populations considered severely ill, including those with psychosis, and have effects on all psychiatric domains, not just those more typically associated with trauma (de Bont et al., 2016; Swan, Keen, Reynolds, & Onwumere, 2017). And so, focusing on the unique meaning and coping tools any given person presents with and understanding it all in the context of one's life may be more important than any given theoretical framework.

In general, according to individuals with lived experience, working with people is an art, not a science (e.g., Smedslund, 2016), and cannot conform to any standardized method of intervention. And, there is no one-sized prescription that dictates there is any specific order in which any of this work take place; for some, working on coping skills and decreasing "symptoms" before any discussion of their feelings or the past is, indeed, necessary. Others, however, find that building relationships and meaning in the present, learning to tolerate their feelings while incorporating some work on coping skills throughout is most helpful. And, because clients of all backgrounds are so easily influenced by authority, allowing the work to be client-led is imperative.

At the same time, there do appear to be some more formalized treatments that are non-pathologizing and do consider many of the above principles that participants, service users, and advocates have found helpful. These include Open Dialogue, IFS, EMDR, somatic therapies, the Maastricht approach and, as was already recommended by standard guidelines, relationship-focused psychodynamic approaches. All of these include the need for learning better coping skills, relationship-building skills, and decreased distress.

Open Dialogue

Open Dialogue (Seikkula, Alakare, & Aaltonen, 2011) is an approach to psychiatric crises, most notably those described as psychotic, that began in Western Lapland, England. The philosophy behind this approach has been expanding in practices, including in the United States (Gordon, Gidugu, Rogers, DeRonck, & Ziedonis, 2016), though in Lapland it is *the* first-line community-wide approach. Open Dialogue is predicated on the idea that collaboration, genuine curiosity and listening, and egalitarianism are central components of care. It does not rely on psychiatric drugs or hospitalization, and drugs are only implemented after a lapse of time exhausting all other measures. Even in these instances, they are used in the smallest doses possible, and often only during the crisis (as opposed to ongoing "maintenance" prescriptions in high doses, as is standard in most of Western medicine).

Typically, when a crisis call comes in, a response will be given within 24 hours. All meetings take place with the person in crisis present, as well as any family members; there are no behind-closed-doors treatment team meetings or decisions made without the individual involved. Uncertainty and flexibility are embraced and a sense of *being with*, rather than *doing to*, is created. The dialogue across meetings and treatment encounters is about truly listening, rather than interpretation or telling the person what he or she should or should not be doing/saying/thinking/and so on.

The goal is not to eradicate "symptoms", but rather to attend to the needs of the whole person, which is not always clear from the outset. Studies have indicated that an Open Dialogue approach results in a reduction in the use of hospitalizations, long-term psychiatric drugs, duration of crisis, need for disability, and overall dysfunction (Lakeman, 2014; Seikkula et al., 2006). This approach appears to have the highest recovery rates in the world from extreme emotional states (Seikkula et al., 2011), providing evidence for the profound effectiveness of a non-authoritarian, egalitarian, collaborative approach to emotional distress that tolerates ambiguity and uncertainty and works with, rather than trying to fix, the person in need. Not only do they have a recovery rate of close to 80% for psychosis, but Open Dialogue operates without diagnoses. While this approach is largely specific to experiences framed as psychotic, it may also be promising for all forms of emotional distress and healing, particularly when considering how it fits with what so many service users are asking for.

Internal Family Systems

One specific form of therapeutic intervention that participants found to be particularly helpful, if used in a flexible and collaborative manner, was the Internal Family Systems (IFS; also discussed in depth in Chap. 5) approach. This approach is part of an overall eclectic treatment plan that may include family therapy, aspects of cognitive therapy, and psychodynamic principles. It is thought of as a metaphorical framework for working collaboratively with the client and respecting his or her beliefs regarding parts of the self (Deacon & Davis, 2001; Goulding & Schwartz, 1995). The goal of IFS is to help the various parts of the self to release their extreme and polarized roles, working more in collaboration and agreement (Pais, 2009). Integration is not a goal, for it is believed that everyone has an internal system of different parts (Schwartz, 1995). Instead the goal is to find balance and harmony within this internal family. This approach may also be useful to address the internal conflicts of a person who is perceived as "psychotic" or "bipolar" versus "dissociative" when looking through a trauma lens (e.g., Bransford & Blizard, 2017; Goldman, 2006). In fact, IFS is non-diagnostic and assumes that all humans consist of multiple parts that are in conflict as a matter of degree. Personally, though I do not utilize formal IFS in my own clinical work, it is quite common for me to incorporate parts work with many of my clients as a means of finding compassion, forgiveness, conflict resolution, awareness, and acceptance for oneself. It is a useful approach regardless of diagnosis, presentation, or level of functioning.

IFS treatment consists of developing insight wherein the individual can differentiate a core Self that can take on the role of therapist in respect to the other parts (Pais, 2009). The role of the therapist in facilitating internal communication and harmony is considered secondary to individuals learning to explore their own internal worlds and interacting with their various parts. Deacon and Davis (2001) outline several techniques that are derived from family therapy and some that are reminiscent of Gestalt therapy (see Fagan & Shepherd, 1970). These techniques include imagery and "open-chair" exercises that facilitate dialogue among parts of the self. Clients may be asked to make "sculptures" of their internal parts and their relationships, using objects in the room, furniture, and so on. These sculptures may be altered over various sessions, boundaries may be physically created, dialogue may be created, and the role of any one part may be physically enacted by the client. Solution-focused questioning may be included in order to help the person to focus on strengths and discover times when the parts were in harmony or balance. The client may be asked to imagine that a miracle occurred and a particular problem was resolved. The therapist would then ask the person to imagine how the parts worked together in bringing about this resolution. Clients may also be asked to role-play interactions between specific parts to resolve conflicts and gain insight to the different perspectives of parts. This allows the person to increase empathy, gain understanding of the original trauma, and learn to distinguish differences between the parts and internalized aspects of significant others (often the abuser). These techniques also allow for explorations of ways in which the therapist's parts are possibly creating problems within the therapy (Miller, Cardona, & Hardin, 2007).

The Maastricht Approach to Hearing Voices

Voice-hearing is increasingly being considered a dissociative experience and possibly a form of expression of dissociated parts of the self (e.g., Pilton, Varese, Berry, & Bucci, 2015). Within this theoretical perspective, IFS and other methods of working with parts of the self can be useful in working with voices. Similar to these approaches, Marius Romme and Sandra Escher (2000), who were fundamental in the formation of the Hearing Voices Network (discussed further in Chap. 9), developed a form of voice dialoguing called the Maastricht approach. It is based on the premise that voices are functional (rather than "symptoms" of an "illness") and need to be understood in order to better understand the internal conflicts and emotions of the whole person. Voices are invited to communicate directly with the therapist, may be mapped out with a strategy formed collaboratively as to an order of engagement, and are valued for the roles they play, rather than dismissed or ignored (see Corstens, Escher, & Romme, 2008 for a summary). Akin to the other approaches discussed thus far, the therapist/client relationship is a primary tool of healing, collaboration is essential, and goals of increased understanding, harmony, and meaning-making are central.

Other Alternative Psychotherapeutic Interventions

In addition to these broader frameworks, there are several adjunctive approaches that can be incorporated and that many service users find useful. EMDR, for instance, may be a more tolerable way of exploring traumatic memories and integrating these experiences into a meaningful narrative than direct verbal exploration. Shapiro (2001) suggest, however, that EMDR only be used with very specific individuals who are higher functioning and by practitioners with in-depth training working with severe dissociation. Other techniques include sensorimotor psychotherapy (Ogden, Minton, & Pain, 2006), expressive therapies (including art and drama therapy), and, for some, short-term use of psychotropic drugs for overt and/or intense experiences that make functioning difficult (Ross, 2007; Van der Kolk, 2014). Van der Kolk (2006) suggests that most psychological trauma-based treatments are overly focused on rational, verbal, cognitive aspects of traumatic memory at the expense of a more bottom-up approach. He asserts that body work and sensorimotor techniques are vital in understanding body memoires that are expressed somatically and in learning to name and tolerate these sensations (van der Kolk, McFarlane, & Welsaeth, 1999).

General exercise has been shown to reduce PTSD and depressive distress (Rosenbaum, Sherrington, & Tiedemann, 2015). Also, family therapy with non-abusive family members can be helpful in assisting with emotional support, mapping of the internal system, and relapse prevention (Pais, 2009). Lastly, narrative therapy is often incorporated as a way to allow people to create autobiographical stories that can be modified throughout the healing process (Miller et al., 2007).

In addition to these more accepted adjunctive practices, hypnosis is often used with complex trauma survivors for the purpose of helping build ego strength (Steele et al., 2005), to identify the traumatic origin of so-called psychotic ideation (van der Hart, Witztum, & Friedman, 1993), to decrease anxiety and other posttraumatic reactions (Cardena, Van Duijl, Weiner, & Terhune, 2009), to access "alters" (Howell, 2011), and to assist in the synthesis and integration of dissociated self-states (van der Hart et al., 2006). It is also used to control and contain intense emotions related to processing of traumatic memories (Steele et al., 2005), as well as subduing aggressive parts of the personality (Ross & Gahan, 1988). At the same time, the search for suspected hidden memories or trying to access "alters" has been greatly criticized for creating inaccurate memories, increased dysfunction and dissociation, and overt manifestation of "personalities" (e.g., Piper & Merskey, 2005; Powell & Gee, 1999; Spanos, 1994, 1996).

Since the time of Pierre Janet, hypnosis has been at the center of a great deal of controversy due to the risk of distorted memories, exaggerated and flamboyant presentations of "multiple personalities", and increased dysfunction. It also may be that the harm in DID-specific treatments, more generally, come more from clinicians who become overly focused on the fantastical aspects of behavior at the expense of working on the client's conflicts and suffering (Chitalkar, Pande, & Shetty, 1996; Gleaves, 1996; Shusta-Hochberg, 2004). Of course, this same criticism could be said about all specialty areas of mental health, perhaps most notably with people diagnosed with psychotic or bipolar disorders. As stated by Harold Searles over half a century ago, in the context of schizophrenia, "A patient cannot identify with a therapist who is running off in all directions after the patient's various personality fragments; instead, the therapist will find that, very frequently, the most useful move is to 'stay put' psychologically, simply acknowledging the feeling or feelings which the patient is endeavouring to convey" (Searles, 1965/1986, p. 398).

NOTE

1. See Hunter and Barsky (2016) for an analysis of the ways in which clinicians, with their particular backgrounds and even traumatic experiences, may clash with the people they are working with in terms of protective worldviews. Existential anxiety, fears of death, meaning-making frameworks, and anxiety stemming from uncertainty are universal experiences. This clash of worldviews or meaning-making systems might be most evident when looking at polarized political or religious factions. This same dynamic appears to exist, quite often, in the professional-client relationship, with very different life experiences leading to rival ideologies that both threaten the other.

REFERENCES

APA Working Group on Investigation of Memories of Childhood Abuse. (1998). First report of the American Psychological Association Working Group on investigation of memories of childhood abuse: Final conclusions of the American Psychological Association Working Group on investigation of memories of childhood abuse. *Psychology, Public Policy and Law, 4,* 931–1306.

Ardito, R. B., & Rabellino, D. (2011). Therapeutic alliance and outcome of psychotherapy: Historical excursus, measurements, and prospects for research. *Frontiers in Psychology, 2,* 270. https://doi.org/10.3389/fpsyg.2011.00270

Bacon, T., & Kennedy, A. (2015). Clinical perspectives on the relationship between psychosis and dissociation: Utility of structural dissociation and implications for practice. *Psychosis, 7*(1), 81–91.

Baker, H., & Baker, N. (1987). Heinz Kohut's self psychology. An overview. *The American Journal of Psychology, 144*(1), 1–9.

Barch, D. M., Bustillo, J., Gaebel, W., Gur, R., Heckers, S., Malaspina, D., … Carpenter, W. (2013). Logic and justification for dimensional assessment of symptoms and related clinical phenomena in psychosis: Relevance to DSM-5. *Schizophr Res, 150*(1), 15–20.

Bentall, R. P. (2003). *Madness explained: Psychosis and human nature.* London: Penguin.

Bjornestad, J., Bronnick, K., Davidson, L., Hegelstad, W. T. V., Joa, I., Kandal, O., … Johannessen, J. O. (2017). The central role of self-agency in clinical recovery from first episode psychosis. *Psychosis, 9*(2), 140–148. https://doi.org/10.1080/17522439.2016.1198828

Blanchard, M., & Farber, B. A. (2016). Lying in psychotherapy: Why and what clients don't tell their therapist about therapy and their relationship. *Counselling Psychology Quarterly, 29*(1), 90–112.

Boevink, W., & Corstens, D. (2012). My body remembers; I refused: Childhood trauma, dissociation and psychosis. In J. Geekie, D. Randal, D. Lampshire, & J. Read (Eds.), *Experiencing Psychosis* (pp. 119–126). New York: Routledge.

Brand, B. L., Classen, C. C., Lanius, R., Loewenstein, R. J., McNary, S. W., Pain, C., & Putnam, F. W. (2009). A naturalistic study of dissociative identity disorder and dissociative disorder nt otherwise specified patients treated by community clinicians. *Psychological Trauma: Theory, Research, Practice, and Policy, 1*(2), 153–171.

Brand, B. L., Classen, C. C., McNary, S. W., & Zaveri, P. (2009). A review of dissociative disorders treatment studies. *Journal of Nervous and Mental Disease, 197*, 646–654.

Brand, B. L., Lanius, R., Vermetten, E., Loewenstein, R. J., & Spiegel, D. (2012). Where are we going? An update on assessment, treatment, and neurobiological research in dissociative disorders as we move toward the DSM-5. *Journal of Trauma & Dissociation, 13*(1), 9–31.

Bransford, C. L., & Blizard, R. A. (2017). Viewing psychopathology through a trauma lens. *Social Work in Mental Health, 15*(1), 80–98. https://doi.org/10.1080/15332985.2016.1173161

Bromberg, P. M. (1995). Resistance, object usage, and human relatedness. *Contemporary Psychoanalysis, 31*(2), 173–191.

Bromberg, P. M. (1998). *Standing in the spaces: Essays on clinical process, trauma, and dissociation.* Hillsdale, NJ: The Analytic Press.

Byrne, R., & Morrison, A. P. (2014). Service users' priorities and preferences for treatment of psychosis: A user-led Delphi study. *Psychiatric Services, 65,* 1167–1169.

Cardena, E., Van Duijl, M., Weiner, L., & Terhune, D. (2009). Possession/trance phenomena. In P. F. Dell & J. A. O'Neil (Eds.), *Dissociation and the Dissociative Disorders: DSM-V and Beyond* (pp. 171–181). New York, NY: Routledge.

Chitalkar, Y., Pande, N., & Shetty, J. (1996). Collusion and entanglement in the therapy of a patient with multiple personalities. *American Journal of Psychotherapy, 50*(2), 243–251.

Cloitre, M., Courtois, C. A., Ford, J. D., Green, B., Alexander, P., Briere, J., … van der Hart, O. (2012). The ISTSS expert consensus treatment guidelines for complex PTSD in adults. Retrieved from https://www.istss.org/ISTSS_Main/media/Documents/ISTSS-Expert-Concesnsus-Guidelines-for-Complex-PTSD-Updated-060315.pdf

Cohen, O. (2005). How do we recover? An analysis of psychiatric survivor oral histories. *Journal of Humanistic Psychology, 45*(3), 333–354.

Connor, K. O., Nelson, B., Walterfang, M., Velakoulis, D., & Thompson, A. (2009). Pseudoneurotic schizophrenia revisited. *Australian and New Zealand Journal of Psychiatry, 43*(9), 873–876.

Coons, P. M., & Bowman, E. A. S. (2001). Ten-year follow-up study of patients with dissociative identity disorder. *Journal of Trauma & Dissociation, 2*(1), 73–89.

Corstens, D., Escher, S., & Romme, M. (2008). Accepting and working with voices: The Maastricht approach. In A. Moskowitz, I. Schafer, & M. J. Dorahy (Eds.), *Psychosis, trauma and dissociation: Emerging perspectives on severe psychopathology* (pp. 319–332). Chichester: Wiley-Blackwell.

Courtois, C. A. (2004). Complex trauma, complex reactions: Assessment and treatment. *Psychotherapy: Theory, Research, Practice, Training, 41*(4), 412–425.

Coyle, T. N., Shaver, J. A., & Linehan, M. M. (2018). On the potential for iatrogenic effects of psychiatric crisis services: The example of dialectical behavior therapy for adult women with borderline personality disorder. *Journal of Consulting and Clinical Psychology, 86*(2), 116–124. https://doi.org/10.1037/ccp0000275

Davies, J. M. (1996). Dissociation, repression and reality testing in the countertransference: The controversey over memory and false memory in the psychoanalytic treatment of adult survivors of childhood sexual abuse. *Psychoanalytic Dialogues, 6*(2), 189–218.

Davies, J. M., & Frawley, M. G. (1991). Dissociative processes and transference-countertransference paradigms in the psychoanalytically oriented treatment of adult survivors of childhood sexual abuse. *Psychoanalytic Dialogues, 2*, 5–36.

de Bont, P. A. J. M., van den Berg, D. P. G., van der Vleugel, B. M., de Roos, C., de Jongh, A., van der Gaag, M., & van Minnen, A. M. (2016). Prolonged exposure and EMDR for PTSD v. a PTSD waiting-list condition: Effects on symptoms of psychosis, depression and social functioning in patients with chronic psychotic disorders. *Psychological Medicine, 46*(11), 2411–2421. https://doi.org/10.1017/s0033291716001094

Deacon, S. A., & Davis, J. C. (2001). Internal family systems theory: A technical integration. *Journal of Systemic Therapies, 20*(1), 45–58.

Dinniss, S., Roberts, G., Hubbard, C., Hounsell, J., & Webb, R. (2007). User-led assessment of a recovery service using DREEM. *The Psychiatrist, 31*(4), 124–127.

Duncan, B. L., Miller, S. D., & Sparks, J. A. (2004). *The heroic client: A revolutionary way to improve effectiveness through client-directed, outcome-informed therapy* (Rev. ed.). San Francisco, CA: John Wiley & Sons, Inc.

Ellason, J. W., & Ross, C. A. (1997). Two-year follow-up of inpatients with dissociative identity disorder. *American Journal of Psychiatry, 154*(6), 832–839.

Fagan, J., & Shepherd, I. L. (1970). *Gestalt therapy now: Theory, techniques, applications*. Oxford: Science & Behavior Books.

Faria, V., Gingnell, M., Hoppe, J. M., Hjorth, O., Alaie, I., Frick, A., ... Furmark, T. (2017). Do you believe it? Verbal suggestions influence the clinical and neural effects of escitalopram in social anxiety disorder: A randomized trial. *EBioMedicine, 24*, 179–188. https://doi.org/10.1016/j.ebiom.2017.09.031

Farkas, M. (2007). The vision of recovery today: What it is and what it means for services. *World Psychiatry, 6,* 4–10.

Fluckiger, C., Del Re, A. C., Wampold, B. E., Symonds, D., & Horvath, A. O. (2012). How central is the alliance in psychotherapy? A multilevel longitudinal meta-analysis. *Journal of Counseling Psychology, 59,* 10–17.

Foley, G. N., & Gentile, J. P. (2010). Nonverbal Communication in Psychotherapy. *Psychiatry (Edgmont), 7*(6), 38–44.

Fonagy, P. (2015). The effectiveness of psychodynamic psychotherapies: An update. *World Psychiatry, 14*(2), 137–150. https://doi.org/10.1002/wps.20235

Freyd, J. J. (1994). Betrayal trauma: Traumatic amnesia as an adaptive response to childhood abuse. *Ethics & Behavior, 4*(4), 307–329.

Gainer, K. (1994). Dissociation and schizophrenia: An historical review of conceptual development and relevant treatment approaches. *Dissociation, 7*(4), 261–271.

Galbusera, L., & Kyselo, M. (2017). The difference that makes the difference: A conceptual analysis of the open dialogue approach. *Psychosis,* 1–8. https://doi.org/10.1080/17522439.2017.1397734

Geekie, J., & Read, J. (2009). *Making sense of madness.* New York: Routledge.

Gibson, S., Brand, S. L., Burt, S., Boden, Z. V., & Benson, O. (2013). Understanding treatment non-adherence in schizophrenia and bipolar disorder: A survey of what service users do and why. *BMC Psychiatry, 13*(1), 153.

Gleaves, D. H. (1996). The sociocognitive model of dissociative identity disorder: A reexamination of the evidence. *Psychological Bulletin, 120*(1), 42–59.

Goldman, I. (2006). IFS: A non-pathologizing approach to mental illness – A personal journey. *Journal of Self Leadership, 2,* 67–71.

Gordon, C., Gidugu, V., Rogers, E. S., DeRonck, J., & Ziedonis, D. (2016). Adapting open dialogue for early-onset psychosis into the U.S. health care environment: A feasibility study. *Psychiatric Services, 67*(11), 1166–1168.

Goulding, R. A., & Schwartz, R. C. (1995). *The mosaic mind: Empowering the tormented selves of child abuse survivors.* New York, NY: W. W. Norton & Company.

Greville-Harris, M., & Dieppe, P. (2015). Bad is more powerful than good: The nocebo response in medical consultations. *The American Journal of Medicine, 128*(2), 126–129.

Harper, S. (2011). An examination of structural dissociation of the personality and the implications for cognitive behavioural therapy. *The Cognitive Behaviour Therapist, 4,* 53–67.

Hawton, K., Witt, K. G., Taylor Salisbury, T. L., Arensman, E., Gunnell, D., Hazell, P., ... van Heeringen, K. (2016). Psychosocial interventions for self-harm in adults. *Cochrane Database of Systematic Reviews, 5.* https://doi.org/10.1002/14651858.cd012189

Hegeman, E. (2009). One or many? Commentary on paper by Debra Rothschild. *Psychoanalytic Dialogues, 19,* 188–196.

Hjorthoj, C. R., Madsen, T., Agerbo, E., & Nordentoft, M. (2014). Risk of suicide according to level of psychiatric treatment: A nationwide nested case-control study. *Social Psychiatry and Psychiatric Epidemiology, 49,* 1357–1365.

Howell, E. (2011). *Understanding and treating dissociative identity disorder: A relational approach.* New York, NY: Taylor and Francis Group, LLC.

Hunter, N., & Barsky, T. V. (2016). Transactional experiences of existential anxiety as a barrier to effective humanistic intervention. *Journal of Humanistic Psychology.* https://doi.org/10.1177/0022167816646671

International Society for the Study of Trauma and Dissociation. (2011). Guidelines for treating dissociative identity disorder in adults, third revision. [Practice Guideline]. *Journal of Trauma & Dissociation, 12*(2), 115–187.

Johnstone, L. (2014). *A straight talking introduction to psychiatric diagnosis.* Monmouth: PCCS Books Ltd.

Johnstone, L. (2017). Psychological formulation as an alternative to psychiatric diagnosis. *Journal of Humanistic Psychology, 58*(1), 30–46.

Johnstone, L., Boyle, M., with Cromby, J., Dillon, J., Harper, D., Kinderman, P., ... Read, J. (2018). The power threat meaning framework: Towards the identification of patterns in emotional distress, unusual experiences and troubled or troubling behaviour, as an alternative to functional psychiatric diagnosis. Retrieved from https://www.bps.org.uk/news-and-policy/introducing-power-threat-meaning-framework

Karon, B. P. (2003). The tragedy of schizophrenia without psychotherapy. *The Journal of the American Academy of Psychoanalysis and Dynamic Psychiatry, 31,* 89–118.

Kernberg, O. F. (1976). *Object relations theory and clinical psychoanalysis.* New York: Aronson.

Kirshner, L. A. (2015). Trauma and psychosis: A review and framework for psychoanalytic understanding. *International Forum of Psychoanalysis, 24*(4), 216–224. https://doi.org/10.1080/0803706x.2013.778422

Kluft, R. P. (2001). The difficult to treat patient with a dissociative disorder. In M. J. Dewan & R. W. Pies (Eds.), *The difficult-to-treat psychiatric patient* (pp. 209–242). Arlington, VA: American Psychiatric Publishing, Inc.

Kohut, H. (1977). *The restoration of the self.* New York: International Universities Press.

Koriat, A., Goldsmith, M., & Pansky, A. (2000). Toward a psychology of memory accuracy. *Annual Review of Psychology, 51,* 481–537.

Kurzban, R. (2010). *Why everyone (else) is a hypocrite.* Princeton, NJ: Princeton University Press.

Lakeman, R. (2014). The Finnish open dialogue approach to crisis intervention in psychosis: A review. *Psychotherapy in Australia, 20*(3), 26–33.

Leichsenring, F., & Steinert, C. (2017). Is cognitive behavioral therapy the gold standard for psychotherapy? The need for plurality in treatment and research. *JAMA, 318*(14), 1323–1324.

McEnteggart, C., Barnes-Holmes, Y., Dillon, J., Egger, J., & Oliver, J. E. (2017). Hearing voices, dissociation, and the self: A functional-analytic perspective. *Journal of Trauma & Dissociation, 18*(4), 575–594.

McHugh, R. K., Whitton, S. W., Peckham, A. D., Welge, J. A., & Otto, M. W. (2013). Patient preference for psychological vs. pharmacologic treatment of psychiatric disorders: A meta-analytic review. *Journal of Clinical Psychiatry, 74*(6), 595–602.

McKenna, P. J., & Kingdon, D. G. (2014). Has cognitive behavioural therapy for psychosis been oversold? *BMJ: British Medical Journal, 348.* https://doi.org/10.1136/bmj.g2295

Mead, S., & Copeland, M. E. (2000). What recovery means to us: Consumers' perspectives. *Community Mental Health Journal, 36*(3), 315–328.

Mehl-Madrona, L., Jul, E., & Mainguy, B. (2014). Results of a transpersonal, narrative, and phenomenological psychotherapy for psychosis. *International Journal of Transpersonal Studies, 33*(1), 57–76.

Miller, B. J., Cardona, J. R. P., & Hardin, M. (2007). The use of narrative therapy and internal family systems with survivors of childhood sexual abuse. *Journal of Feminist Family Therapy, 18*(4), 1–27.

Modell, A. H. (2005). Emotional memory, metaphor, and meaning. *Psychoanalytic Inquiry, 25*(4), 555–568.

Morrison, A. P. (2001). The interpretation of intrusions in psychosis: An integrative cognitive approach to psychotic symptoms. *Behavioural & Cognitive Psychotherapy, 29,* 257–276.

Morrison, A. P. (2009). A cognitive behavioural perspective on the relationship between childhood trauma and psychosis. *Epidemiologia e Psichiatria Sociale, 18*(4), 294–298.

Mosquera, D., & Ross, C. A. (2017). A psychotherapy approach to treating hostile voices. *Psychosis, 9*(2), 167–175.

Myrick, A., Brand, B. L., & Putnam, F. W. (2013). For better or worse: The role of revictimization and stress in the courses of treatment for dissociative disorders. *Journal of Trauma & Dissociation, 14,* 375–389.

National Health Service. (2015). *The Five Year Forward View Mental Health Taskforce: Public engagement findings.* London: National Health Service.

Neil, S. T., Kilbride, M., Pitt, L., Nothard, S., Welford, M., Sellwood, W., & Morrison, A. P. (2009). The questionnaire about the process of recovery (QPR): A measurement tool developed in collaboration with service users. *Psychosis, 1*(2), 145–155.

Ogden, P., Minton, K., & Pain, C. (2006). *Trauma and the body: A sensorimotor approach to psychotherapy.* New York, NY: W. W. Norton.

Pais, S. (2009). A systematic approach to the treatment of dissociative identity disorder. *Journal of Family Psychotherapy, 20*(1), 72–88.

Pilton, M., Varese, F., Berry, K., & Bucci, S. (2015). The relationship between dissociation and voices: A systematic literature review and meta-analysis. *Clinical Psychology Review, 40*, 138–155.

Piper, A., Jr., & Merskey, H. (2005). Reply: The persistence of folly: A critical examination of dissociative identity disorder. *The Canadian Journal of Psychiatry, 50*(12).

Powell, R. A., & Gee, T. L. (1999). The effects of hypnosis on dissociative identity disorder: A reexamination of the evidence. *Canadian Journal of Psychiatry, 44*, 914–916.

Randal, P., Stewart, M. W., Proverbs, D., Lampshire, D., Symes, J., & Hamer, H. (2009). "The Re-covery Model" – An integrative developmental stress-vulnerability-strengths approach to mental health. *Psychosis, 1*(2), 122–133.

Rogers, C. R. (1961/1995). *On becoming a person: A therapist's view of psychotherapy*. Boston, MA: Houghton Mifflin Company.

Romme, M., & Escher, S. (2000). *Making Sense of Voices*. London: Mind Publications.

Rosenbaum, S., Sherrington, C., & Tiedemann, A. (2015). Exercise augmentation compared with usual care for post-traumatic stress disorder: A randomized controlled trial. *Acta Psychiatrica Scandinavica, 131*(5), 350–359.

Ross, C. A. (2007). *The trauma model: A solution to the problem of comorbidity in psychiatry*. Richardson, TX: Manitou Communications, Inc.

Ross, C. A., & Gahan, P. (1988). Techniques in the treatment of multiple personality disorder. *American Journal of Psychotherapy, 42*(1), 40–52.

Ross, C. A., & Keyes, B. (2004). Dissociation and schizophrenia. *Journal of Trauma & Dissociation, 5*(3), 69–83.

Schwartz, R. C. (1995). *Internal family systems therapy*. New York: Guilford.

Scoboria, A., Mazzoni, G., Kirsch, I., & Milling, L. S. (2002). Immediate and persisting effects of misleading questions and hypnosis on memory reports. *Journal of Experimental Psychology, 8*, 26–32.

Searles, H. F. (1965/1986). *Collected papers on schizophrenia and related subjects* (Reprint ed.). London: Karnac Books Ltd.

Seikkula, J., Aaltonen, J., Alakare, B., Haarakangas, K., Keranen, J., & Lehtinen, K. (2006). Five-year experience of first-episode nonaffective psychosis in open-dialogue approach: Treatment principles, follow-up outcomes, and two case studies. *Psychotherapy Research, 16*(2), 214–228.

Seikkula, J., Alakare, B., & Aaltonen, J. (2011). The comprehensive open-dialogue approach in Western Lapland: II. Long-term stability of acute psychosis outcomes in advanced community care. *Psychosis, 3*, 192–204.

Shapiro, F. (2001). *Eye movement desensitization and reprocessing: Basic principles, protocols and procedures* (2nd ed.). New York, NY: Guilford Press.

Shedler, J. (2015). Where is the evidence for "evidence-based" therapy? *The Journal of Psychological Therapies in Primary Care, 4*, 47–59.

Shumway, M., Saunders, T., Shern, D., Pines, E., Downs, A., Burbine, T., & Beller, J. (2003). Preferences for schizophrenia treatment outcomes among public policy makers, consumers, families, and providers. *Psychiatric Services, 54*, 1124–1128.

Shusta-Hochberg, S. R. (2004). Therapeutic hazards of treating child alters as real children in dissociative identity disorder. *Journal of Trauma & Dissociation, 5*(1), 13–27.

Silver, A.-L. S. (2003). The psychotherapy of schizophrenia: It's place in the modern world. *The Journal of the American Academy of Psychoanalysis and Dynamic Psychiatry, 31*(2), 325–342.

Sinason, V., & Silver, A.-L. S. (2008). Treating dissociative and psychotic disorders psychodynamically. In A. Moskowitz, I. Schafer, & M. J. Dorahy (Eds.), *Psychosis, trauma and dissociation: Emerging perspectives on severe psychopathology* (pp. 239–254). West Sussex: John Wiley and Sons, Ltd.

Smedslund, J. (2016). Why psychology cannot be an empirical science. *Integrative Psychological and Behavioral Science, 50*(2), 185–195.

Spanos, N. P. (1994). Multiple identity enactments and multiple personality disorder: A sociocognitive perspective. *Psychological Bulletin, 116*(1), 143–165.

Spanos, N. P. (1996). *Multiple identities and false memories*. Washington, DC: American Psychological Association.

Steele, K., & van der Hart, O. (2009). Treating dissociation. In C. A. Courtois & J. D. Ford (Eds.), *Treating complex traumatic stress disorder*. New York: Guilford Press.

Steele, K., van der Hart, O., & Nijenhuis, E. R. (2001). Dependency in the treatment of complex posttraumatic stress disorder and dissociative disorders. *Journal of Trauma & Dissociation, 2*(4), 79–116.

Steele, K., van der Hart, O., & Nijenhuis, E. R. (2005). Phase-oriented treatment of structural dissociation in complex traumatization: Overcoming trauma-related phobias. *Journal of Trauma & Dissociation, 6*, 11–53.

Steinert, C., Munder, T., Rabung, S., Hoyer, J., & Falk, L. (2017). Psychodynamic therapy: As efficacious as other empirically supported treatments? A meta-analysis testing equivalence of outcomes. *The American Journal of Psychiatry, 174*(10), 943–953.

Stern, D. B. (2004). The eye sees itself: Dissociation, enactment, and the achievement of conflict. *Contemporary Psychoanalysis, 40*, 197–237.

Swan, S., Keen, N., Reynolds, N., & Onwumere, J. (2017). Psychological interventions for post-traumatic stress symptoms in psychosis: A systematic review of outcomes. *Frontiers in Psychology, 8*(341). https://doi.org/10.3389/fpsyg.2017.00341

Swift, J. K., Tompkins, K. A., & Parkin, S. R. (2017). Understanding the client's perspective of helpful and hindering events in psychotherapy sessions: A micro-process approach. *Journal of Clinical Psychology, 73*(11), 1543–1555. https://doi.org/10.1002/jclp.22531

The British Psychological Society. (2014). *Guidelines on language in relation to functional psychiatric diagnosis.* Leicester: The British Psychological Society.

Topor, A., & Denhov, A. (2015). Going beyond: Users' experiences of helping professionals. *Psychosis, 7*(3), 228–236.

Tuttman, S. (1990). Exploring an object relations perspective on borderline conditions. *Journal of the American Academy of Psychoanalysis, 18*(4), 539–553.

van der Hart, O., Nijenhuis, E. R., & Steele, K. (2006). *The haunted self: Structural dissociation and the treatment of chronic traumatization.* New York, NY: W. W. Norton.

van der Hart, O., Witztum, E., & Friedman, B. (1993). From hysterical psychosis to reactive dissociative psychosis. *Journal of Traumatic Stress, 6*(1), 43–64.

van der Kolk, B. A. (1989). The compulsion to repeat the trauma. *Psychiatric Clinics of North America, 12*(2), 389–411.

van der Kolk, B. A. (2006). Clinical implications of neuroscience research in PTSD. *Annals of the New York Academy of Sciences, 1070,* 277–293.

van der Kolk, B. A. (2014). *The body keeps the score: Brain, mind, and body in the healing of trauma.* New York, NY: Penguin Books.

van der Kolk, B. A., McFarlane, A. C., & Welsaeth, L. (1999). *Traumatic stress: Effects of overwhelming experience on mind, body and society.* New York: Guilford Press.

Varese, F., Udachina, A., Myin-Germeys, I., Oorschot, M., & Bentall, R. P. (2011). The relationship between dissociation and auditory verbal hallucinations in the flow of daily life of patients with psychosis. *Psychosis, 3*(1), 14–28.

Williams, P. (2012). *Rethinking madness: Towards a paradigm shift in our understanding and treatment of psychosis.* San Rafael, CA: Sky's Edge Publishing.

Williamson, C. (2009). The patient movement as an emancipation movement. *Health Expectations, 11,* 102–112.

Winnicott, D. W. (1965/1990). *The maturational process and the facilitating environment.* London: Karnac.

Zilcha-Mano, S., Roose, S. P., Barber, J. P., & Rutherford, B. R. (2015). Therapeutic alliance in antidepressant treatment: Cause or effect of symptomatic levels? *Psychotherapy and Psychosomatics, 84*(3), 177–182. https://doi.org/10.1159/000379756

CHAPTER 8

A Plea for Change

It's kind of like we all get this kind of script that 'this is what you do when you're a professional working with people.' It's all to me bullshit. It's nice to know some of it though. I think it can help. However, I still think it's bullshit. I think it's just, ya know, when somebody has it more genuine, where it's in their character. P10

The problems inherent in medicalized formulations and treatment of emotional distress and the sometimes paternalistic, authoritarian behavior of mental health professionals are consistently criticized by individuals with lived experience, and all of the participants, to be harmful and re-traumatizing (Boevink, 2012; Cohen, 2005; Dillon, 2013; Gibson, Brand, Burt, Boden, & Benson, 2013; McHugh, Whitton, Peckham, Welge, & Otto, 2013; Mead & Copeland, 2000; Thomas & Longden, 2013). This includes the use of multiple, high-dose psychotropic drugs, forced hospitalizations, compulsory "treatment" orders in the community, medicalized language and framing of emotional experience, coercive behaviors and judgments, and so on. Service users describe experiences of force and coercion in mental health services as akin to imprisonment, being ambushed, and feeling terrorized (e.g., Murphy et al., 2017) at a most vulnerable time of life.

Individuals experiencing psychological or spiritual crises often describe this period as one fueled by a search for meaning and purpose (e.g., Corin, Thara, & Padmavati, 2004). Telling a person who is searching for meaning and attempting to overcome trauma that their perspectives or narratives

© The Author(s) 2018   183
N. Hunter, *Trauma and Madness in Mental Health Services*,
https://doi.org/10.1007/978-3-319-91752-8_8

are simply wrong, or, worse, delusional, is invalidating and harmful. At the same time, as discussed in Chap. 7, a balance between validating a person's subjective experience and gently challenging and/or reframing their beliefs over time can be found when there is trust, mutuality, and collaboration. The system as a whole, however, is not built on a respect for the subjective and experience-based expertise of the service user; rather, it is predicated on an authoritarian form of social control and coercive practices. Advocates and service users continue to plead for change, with the UN Special Rapporteur calling for the complete ending of forced treatments throughout the world due to the inhumane and harmful nature of these practices (Mendez, 2013).

Stop Talking About "Symptoms"

I think that people talk in circles about the stigma of mental illness, while we know that when you stop medicalizing people's experiences and look at what happened in that person's life and how these 'symptoms' are serving them, that that's when you have a real chance to help them out. P1

Being on a lot of psychiatric medicine is really harmful I've found, as far as being healed, healing yourself, in therapy, because it just shuts down everything … I didn't progress in therapy at all really because I felt, like, really kind of numb to my feelings. I didn't feel like I needed to work so hard in therapy. I lost my motivation. P3

Any form of treatment that focuses on illness is an issue for me. Basically the entire biochemical model is an issue for me … it's never even so much the specific treatment form as it is the belief system. I know trauma therapists who subscribe to that model, and, ya know being a trauma therapist isn't like a get-out-jail-free card. I don't know how to describe it. I know some horrific trauma therapists. P13

Whether under the umbrella of schizophrenia, DID, bipolar disorder, or BPD, it appears that, in general, people who have experienced extreme states of distress, altered states of consciousness, extrasensory perceptions, and/or suicidality tend to not have a goal of decreasing "symptoms" so much as finding meaning and purpose, building relationships, having one's life experience and trauma recognized and acknowledged, increasing functioning, and decreasing overall distress. People want to be validated, listened to, and seen as a person, not a set of symptoms to be fixed (e.g., see Schizophrenia Commission, 2012). Although some may find diagnoses and other medical frameworks to be helpful, particularly for the perceived explanation they ostensibly provide, overall, making assumptions, focusing on internal defect, taking a top-down expert/patient approach, and stigmatization (all things that are the result of diagnosing and/or medicalizing distress) can be incredibly harmful.

On the other hand, both therapists and service users find benefit in the challenging and time-consuming process of actually connecting "symptoms" to past trauma and adversity (Halpin, Kugathasan, Hulbert, Alvarez-Jimenez, & Bendall, 2016). So-called symptoms not only have meaning, but also may be a necessary survival strategy, even if they may appear destructive to others. Immediately focusing on getting rid of symptoms can be experienced as life-threatening in this circumstance. Wilma Boevink (2006), a person who spent many years as a patient and is now a premier Dutch psychiatric researcher, describes how her so-called symptoms helped her to survive chronic abuse and trauma and, in turn, how treatment perpetuated this trauma much of the time. She argues that "the threat and the betrayal … feed psychosis, excusing the offender and accusing the victim, forcing the child to accept the reality of the adult, distorting reality, forcing you to betray yourself—experiences extended by psychiatry, reinforce the search to be blamed and confirmation of guilt … In becoming a psychiatric patient, we are supported in our belief that we are bad" (p. 18).

Commonly, a first-line approach when working with people in crisis or extreme emotional distress is to strongly suggest, if not insist upon, the use of psychiatric drugs. The complex problems involved with psychotropic drugs and the standard use of them as maintenance measures, as medicines versus drugs, in cocktails, and with force have been discussed at length elsewhere (see, for instance, Gotzsche, 2015; Whitaker, 2010). For some, the use of psychotropic drugs can be helpful, though the effect most often is due to short-term numbing of emotional distress and/or assistance with sleep (Moncrieff, Cohen, & Porter, 2013). At the same time, these numbing effects can prevent a person from fully engaging in the therapeutic process (e.g., Karon, 2000), and from learning or making meaning of experiences. They also may result in avoidance of confronting the psychosocial stressors that led to the emotional distress in the first place. Additionally, some of these drugs may directly induce psychosis and/or mania, increased violence, and increased suicidality (e.g., Breggin, 2008; Healy, 2012; Healy, Herxheimer, & Menkes, 2006). Generally, in opposition to what is usually offered, service users prefer psychological intervention with minimal use of drugs (McHugh et al., 2013).

In addition to psychiatric drugs, electroconvulsive therapy (ECT) is a surprisingly common intervention given to those with prolonged difficulties, often against their will, when the focus is on symptom management or dissipation of emotions. This intervention is most frequently implemented in state hospitals and long-term residential facilities. The idea is that electrocuting the brain will help people to be less depressed or psychotic and that this process will stimulate brain growth. Yet, there is no evidence that ECT is more effective than active placebo (Read & Arnold, 2017). In other words, people are being forcibly electrocuted without evidence that this practice is actually helpful in the long run. Psychologist Craig Newnes (2016) has likened ECT to other assaultive treatments of the past, such as blood-letting, leeches, insulin comas, lobotomy, and forced sterilization. Read and Arnold (2017) argue that this practice is ethically unjustified. Yet, it continues to be widely used, at least in standard practice within the United States, United Kingdom, and other Western cultures.

The difficulties stemming from being prescribed multiple psychotropic drugs and invasive interventions, however, are the result of adhering to a broader medical model that dictates all mental health treatment. As stated by Read (2004), "many [psychiatrists] believe that the medications are treating the symptoms of an illness, rather than tranquilizing people into pacifity and compliance, partly or primarily for the convenience of others" (p. 34). Participants described the invalidation they felt and the associated shame, hopelessness, and lack of agency that came with being told they have a "mental illness". This is particularly harmful when the illness label is one stereotypically considered biological in nature.

The effects are worst when labeled or drugged as a child, especially when active abuse is ignored, intentionally or otherwise, because the child is perceived as having an "illness" instead of displaying understandable reactions to said ignored abuse. Children are often inadvertently complicit in this, as they naturally try to protect their parents and guardians and fear potential consequences. Burstow (2017) has argued that "the psychiatric drugging of children is a form of child abuse" in itself. Many of the participants spoke of how the numbing effects of drugs as children "helped" by allowing them to endure ongoing physical and sexual abuse that was never revealed to mental health professionals.

Participants spoke about fears of child protective services taking them away from their families, being killed by abusive parents, or just facing the reality of being betrayed by a parent who could harm them so profoundly.

Children (and adults) do not want to betray their own parents. And, so, lying or covering up their abusive situations and taking on the sick role become protective measures. Of course, it is not always about overt abuse. Taking on the sick role within the family also allows for an identifiable reason for the child's distress without ever having to address painful, toxic dynamics within the family or problematic situations in the school, such as poor education and bullying.

Illness conceptualizations tend to result in a decreased sense of responsibility and, for some, even an excuse for bad behavior. Blaming or accusing an individual for disturbing behaviors never results in productive changes in behavior or dialogue; taking the time to truly understand the individual's experiences and behaviors in the context in which they developed and exist is crucial. A the same time, some, including several participants, do sometimes assert that if their "symptoms" cause them to do something, then they lack agency and have less motivation to try to control or take responsibility for their behaviors. One participant (8) recognized this, stating that "it made me feel very out of control and as a result I maybe let the idea that I was out of control let my guard down so that I wasn't controlling myself, if that makes sense".

Medicalized frameworks and their associated diagnoses are complex issues. Some find comfort in receiving a label that provides an illusion of explanation, direction, and solidarity with others who may have similar experiences. This is especially true when the diagnosis is one that is associated with acknowledgment of the traumatic etiology, such as DID or PTSD. Nevertheless, it is common practice to make erroneous assumptions based on the labeling of issues with various diagnoses and the prejudice (i.e., "stigma") associated with many of these categories. As stated at length in Chap. 4, diagnoses lack validity and reliability (British Psychological Society, 2013; Deacon, 2013) and instead result in biased heuristics and stereotypical assumptions that are usually untrue and often defeatist. Who would want to accept a medical diagnosis that amounts to calling some a "bitch" (i.e., BPD), as described by P13? Who deserves being given a label that means one's experiences are meaningless symptoms of a life-long deteriorating disease (i.e., schizophrenia), when the actual evidence appears to suggest the opposite (see Chap. 6)? The labeling of psychological problems with some of these diagnoses has been empirically shown to be disastrous for many. For instance, recently being a given diagnosis of schizophrenia appears sufficient to increase the likelihood that someone will complete suicide (Fleischhacker et al., 2014).

Labels are not necessary for recovery, for treatment formulation, nor for finding camaraderie with peers, even if recognition of specific experiences of the individual is. The profiles of people who have experiences that earn them particular labels are extremely varied, so that any two people with same diagnosis may have no overlap in experience at all (Goldberg, 2011; Skodol et al., 2002; Tandon, 2014; van Os, 2016; Wardenaar & de Jonge, 2013)! For example, individuals who get a diagnosis of DID will certainly have in common an internal sense of distinct selves, or people, living inside them along with associated memory difficulties. Beyond this, however, any given individual's specific constellation of difficulties has almost infinite possibilities. Some people may self-harm, some experience altered reality; some experience states commonly referred to as "mania"; some are obsessive and engage in repetitive behaviors; some are severely depressed and immobile; some shut down and become unemotional, even catatonic, while others are hyper-emotional and/or just hyper; some are chronically suicidal; some are anxious and hypervigilant; some are homeless, while others pursue higher education and management positions; some have families, while others are isolated and alone; and some experience all or none of the above at any given time. A diagnostic label and insinuations that any of these experiences are "symptoms" of specific "diseases" obscure these numerous differences and lead to many assumptions that may or may not be true. The common practice of the medical model lends itself to just adding on additional diagnosis after diagnosis to account for these varied presentations, so that individuals with a DID diagnosis, for example, typically end up with an average of seven to ten total diagnoses (Dell, 1998; Ellason, Ross, & Fuchs, 1996). Additionally, these diagnoses and labels perpetuate sexist and racist oppression (Caplan, 1995; Metzl, 2010; Widiger & Spitzer, 1991).

The problems with medical conceptualizations and focusing on symptoms instead of meaning-making and empowerment are harmful and counter-therapeutic. Such practices are based in an ideological paradigm (Chap. 3) that defies much of the accumulated science and leaves people feeling damaged, defective, marginalized, inferior, and unheard. Individuals who have experienced chronic oppression, adversity, and/or trauma, which essentially refers to most people receiving these labels and treatments, too often end up finding themselves in repetitive oppressive and traumatic dynamics with those who are presumably there to help.

I Don't Want to Be Fixed, I'm Not Fragile

A lot of the stuff I've interacted with that has been supposed to be brilliantly helpful for someone like me hasn't [been]. It's been so medical model, so 'you are broken', um, 'you need to be fixed'. P5

It's not all just bleak arduous survival, guys. Survival can be spirited too. Spirited and inspired and if you offer nothing to this then I am surviving you now. P7

I don't see it as about fixing me. I don't think I need to be fixed. P9

I wish they hadn't taken away that process [of self-harm] for me until I could be stabilized and until the trauma was dealt with because I think that's what caused … [my] psychotic break. Just, it was taken from me. It was just ripped … It's just forced, essentially, in a sense. And, I wish people knew just how sensitive it is to take that away from somebody. P13

Inherent in the medical model is the idea that people need to go to an expert, who will treat them and hopefully fix what is broken. Implicit in this idea, of course, is that something within the individual is deficient (i.e., the broken brain). If there was any evidence that this was objectively true, it might not be a problem. But, as discussed at length throughout Chap. 6, this is not necessarily the case. People adapt to the environments in which they develop, and do so in unique ways. There can be much reward in helping people to grow and adapt to new realities through caring, supportive, empowering, respectful, patient, and safe relationships, and therapy can often be a place for this for some people. Participants expressed strongly, however, that they did not view themselves as needing to be fixed because they are not broken or suffering a disease. They are, on the other hand, suffering the results of a harsh and traumatic world and need empathy, support, and validation in order to grow and become valuable contributing members of society, which everyone has the potential to do. From this perspective, doctors are not necessary, even if they can be helpful for some.

An analogy describing the difference can be seen in looking at a car, for instance. If my car has been vandalized and no longer works, I have several options. I could take it to a mechanic (like a doctor) and see if he or she can fix what is wrong internally. Of course, if this mechanic were parallel to a psychiatrist, I would walk away knowing that my car had "does not start disorder" and be told that this is somehow explanatory and helpful. But, I digress. The car may not start or work because, say, a part got knocked out of place in the course of being hurt by some other person.

Now my options include taking the car to a mechanic, a body shop, or getting some knowledgeable friends together to attend to the damage (wounds) done to the car. With some dedication, I also could just care for the car myself. A mechanic (doctor) is not necessary, even if he or she would be useful in some aspects for some people.

Emotional and behavioral difficulties are not fundamentally diseased or "maladaptive", nor does anyone *need* to be fixed by some expert. In fact, as long considered within psychoanalytic frameworks, emotional and behavioral patterns are most often defensive and may help a person to cope with traumatic and extreme circumstances. It is important to have such strengths and the adaptive nature of these processes to be recognized. Having problems does not mean someone has a disease in need of fixing. The creative ways in which one learns to cope with overwhelming experiences may have many benefits, not just deficits or destruction. Insisting or forcing a person to adapt to a world that has historically been harmful by dropping their survival strategies is akin to robbing a bear of its fur and expecting it to live through the winter.

Force and Coercion Are Not Helpful

There needs to be widespread understanding that locking up trauma survivors against their will is, in no way, therapeutic. P1

He was very authoritative ... he does it to us ... our opinion is welcome but irrelevant ... a lot of the rest of the, particularly in the DID field is, it's authoritative, it's problematic. P5

I think with ... the psychologist ... the sessions were so structured ... that I kind of just started to recite everything. Like, I got to the point where I didn't even feel like we were talking about myself. I was just practicing answering questions ... It didn't mean anything to me. P7

I will always be torn now and deeply know that one must enter at one's own risk, because that risk could far outweigh the very issues of what they may think is a problem in their life right now—far more than one could ever imagine and that what ends up being a final result of Hell may never have existed within themselves prior. P10

It usually happens with my psychologist ... I'll get dragged off to the emergency department until I'm more with it and can go home ... It's really, really stressful. Like they'll induce as much pain as they can ... which doesn't work. It just scares them even more. It sucks. P11

The medical professionals, that's what they're doing. At the drop of a hat, they will start these [involuntary commitment] proceedings with no regard for what the best interest of the patient is. P12

It is understood by many professionals that harm may result from forced interventions, particularly involuntary hospitalizations and forced drugging, but often they are invoked under the guise of protection and doing it for one's own good (see, e.g., The Lancet Psychiatry, 2017 for a discussion). People who are presumed to "lack insight" are treated paternalistically and told what they need in order to feel better, and/or are held against their will until they learn to comply and tell the doctors what they want to hear. Rarely are such individuals respected for their unique ways of making sense of unbearable circumstances or internal pain that makes sense in the context of their lives.

Those who voice their desire to die or attempt to kill themselves are also frequently locked up against their will, with the illusion that a proper assessment of risk can predictably save lives. Yet, according to a study by Large and Ryan (2014), there is little evidence that professionals can predict who will or will not die by suicide. Risk scales may actually serve more a purpose of providing a sense of false reassurance to professionals rather than actually help to prevent suicide. While some individuals may, indeed, have been saved by a forced hospitalization, more generally speaking this is not the case; the benefit for a few does not outweigh the harm for the many. On the other hand, treatment on voluntary, unlocked wards compared with forced treatment is actually associated with less chance of someone attempting suicide (Huber et al., 2016). Perhaps most disturbingly, those who are most likely to be detained forcibly are those who are also the most economically and socially disadvantaged in society (McWade, 2016) once again demonstrating the possibly classist and racist dynamics underlying much of standard mental health practices and assumptions.

Force and coercion also include more seemingly benign behaviors on the part of professionals, such as an authoritarian demeanor or attitude and imposing ideas or particular theoretical frameworks onto another's experience. Any goal or framework risks becoming counter-therapeutic and even harmful when it is forced. This includes insisting that individuals conceptualize their experiences in the way that the clinician deems normal or healthy, being overly structured to the point of not listening or being attuned to where the client is at, and/or insisting that the individual define his or her experiences in a manner fitting with the clinicians' theoretical framework rather than honoring the meaning and understanding that makes the most sense to the individual. Considering the central importance of a sense of self-agency and control, accountability, and responsibility in the recovery process (Bjornestad et al., 2017), it is clear that taking such control away and rendering a person helpless to his or her "illness" is not helpful, at best.

More detrimental, however, are forced drugging and hospitalizations, or threats of such. Forced treatment is associated with a poor therapeutic relationship (Hofer, Habermeyer, Mokros, Lau, & Gairing, 2015), which can be particularly damaging bearing in mind that the relationship is a key factor in determining if treatment is actually effective or not. Further, there is evidence that a sense of agency, or control, in one's treatment and life is central to recovery (Bjornestad et al., 2017). It may be taken for granted that individuals who are in acute distress *must* be medicated and that these purported medicines are treating a specific disease process. And, so, if someone refuses to take these drugs, then they *must* be forced to do so for their own good.

Yet, there are several non-medical approaches, such as Open Dialogue (Seikkula, Alakare, & Aaltonen, 2011), that find success with minimal to no use of psychiatric drugs. Psychiatrists in the United Kingdom have urged their colleagues across the globe to be more cautious when prescribing these drugs, and acknowledge that many people can and do recover without the use of psychiatric drugs (e.g., Murray et al., 2016). Not wanting to take these drugs, especially in the long term, is not due to a "lack of insight". People who choose to not take psychiatric drugs beyond an acute crisis period tend to do so because of severe disabling effects of these drugs (see Moore & Furberg, 2017 for a review), with most being satisfied with their decision (Ostrow, Jessell, Hurd, Darrow, & Cohen, 2017). Additionally, those who stop taking these drugs tend to have *higher* rates of long-term recovery than those who do not (Harrow & Jobe, 2007; Harrow, Jobe, & Faull, 2012; Moilanen et al., 2016; Wunderink, Nieboer, Wiersma, Sytema, & Nienhuis, 2013), suggesting that, in fact, the decision to not take drugs may be one that is based on actually having more insight. Even worse, psychotropic drugs have the danger of creating increased mental distress and iatrogenic disability (Lucire, 2016), and service users rarely receive true informed consent or adequate information even when the drugging is not forced (Cartwright, Gibson, Read, Cowan, & Dehar, 2016; Ostrow et al., 2017). Certainly, with fully informed consent, people should have the right to voluntarily take a drug and not be shamed for it if they find it helpful. But, true informed consent is rare, while the benefits of these drugs are regularly exaggerated, especially when being forced.

In addition to the problems with psychiatric drugs, hospitalizations tend to be deemed unhelpful, at best, and traumatizing for many, particularly when they are involuntary. For instance, Mueser, Lu, Rosenberge, and Wolfe (2010) found that over 30% of a patient sample carrying a psychotic diagnosis met full criteria for PTSD as a direct result of their hospital experience. Even for those who might otherwise voluntarily seek help, such commitments often result in people dropping out of therapy altogether and not trusting that they can get help from anybody.

Despite the potential harm that comes from involuntarily detaining a person against his or her will, there is little evidence to support that this is necessary. Studies comparing inpatient hospitalizations to less restrictive care and housing programs consistently fail to demonstrate any superior benefit (Calton, Ferriter, Huband, & Spandler, 2008; Fenton, Mosher, Herrell, & Blyler, 1998; Greenfield, Stoneking, Humphreys, Sundby, & Bond, 2008; Lloyd-Evans, Slade, Jagielska, & Johnson, 2009; Sledge et al., 1996), while the highest rates of completed suicide tend to be *after* discharge from a hospital (Chung et al., 2017). In other words, being imprisoned and forced to get "help" shows no benefit beyond those effects found for people who actually want to be helped, while it does appear to be related to people dying by suicide after they have undergone such "treatment".

In addition to forced hospitalization, perhaps one of the more controversial and possibly harmful forms of force comes in the form of outpatient commitment orders, euphemistically termed "Assisted Outpatient Treatment" in the United States. These are court-ordered mandates for individuals living in the community to comply with "treatment" orders, namely long-term, daily use of psychiatric drugs. Further, for most, noncompliance with such orders may result in loss of housing or disability benefits.

The goal is forced compliance purportedly in an effort to decrease hospitalizations, suicide, violence, relapse, and/or incarceration in jails (as opposed to hospitals). In line with everything discussed thus far, there is a limited and conflicting evidence base to support its use (Rowe, 2013). And, the evidence that does exist is marred by bias and allegiance to ideology (Kisely, Campbell, & Preston, 2011). When such bias is controlled for, however, there is no significance found for hospitalization rates, adherence to treatment, or violent crime (Steadman et al., 2001). In a major Cochrane systematic review on involuntary outpatient commitment (Kisely et al., 2011), the authors concluded that there was no evidence that these orders resulted in any differences in service use, social functioning, or quality of life. Further, it serves to deter those who might otherwise seek voluntary care due to fears of being committed (Allen & Smith, 2001). So, people are being forced to take toxic, deadly drugs that have little evidence of helping long-term in exchange for not being thrown out on the streets and losing whatever meager benefits the government is offering them. All of this in the name of medicine.

The traumatizing nature of forced interventions for innocent people who have committed no crime has been recognized within the United Nations as inhumane and akin to torture (Human Rights Council, 2009). The harm and trauma that results from forced treatment, medicalized conceptualizations of problems, dismissive and authoritarian behaviors from mental health professionals, and the harms from being prescribed multiple psychotropic drugs must be taken seriously by the field as a whole, particularly in light of repeated evidence that increased contact with more restrictive psychiatric interventions is associated, in a dose-response fashion, with an increased rate of completed suicide (Hjorthoj, Madsen, Agerbo, & Nordentoft, 2014; Large & Ryan, 2014). The role of the mental health professionals in providing social control for an over-populated society is also one that must be recognized and not promoted as "treatment". And, of course, professionals need to accept the fact that they are not a necessary part of the healing process, even if they can be extraordinarily helpful for some. Healing comes in many forms, but it rarely results from force, coercion, marginalization, or invalidation of one's life experiences. Punishment rarely begets long-term positive change.

REFERENCES

Allen, M., & Smith, V. F. (2001). Opening pandora's box: The practical and legal dangers of involuntary outpatient commitment. *Psychiatric Services, 52*(3), 342–346.

Bjornestad, J., Bronnick, K., Davidson, L., Hegelstad, W. T. V., Joa, I., Kandal, O., ... Johannessen, J. O. (2017). The central role of self-agency in clinical recovery from first episode psychosis. *Psychosis, 9*(2), 140–148. https://doi.org/10.1080/17522439.2016.1198828

Boevink, W. (2006). From being a disorder to dealing with life: An experiential exploration of the association between trauma and psychosis. *Schizophrenia Bulletin, 32*, 17–19.

Boevink, W. (2012). Towards recovery, empowerment and experiential expertise of users of psychiatric services. In P. Ryan, S. Ramon, & T. Greacen (Eds.),

Empowerment, lifelong learning and recovery in mental health: Towards a new paradigm. New York, NY: Palgrave Macmillan.

Breggin, P. R. (2008). *Medication madness: A psychiatrist exposes the dangers of mood-altering drugs.* New York, NY: St. Martin's Press.

British Psychological Society. (2013). Division of Clinical Psychology position statement on the classification of behaviour and experience in relation to functional psychiatric diagnoses: Time for a paradigm shift. Retrieved from http://dxrevisionwatch.files.wordpress.com/2013/05/position-statement-on-diagnosis-master-doc.pdf

Burstow, B. (2017). Psychiatric drugging of children and youth as a form of child abuse: Not a radical proposition. *Ethical Human Psychology and Psychiatry, 19*(1), 65–76.

Calton, T., Ferriter, M., Huband, N., & Spandler, H. (2008). A systematic review of the soteria paradigm for the treatment of people diagnosed with schizophrenia. *Schizophrenia Bulletin, 34*(1), 181–192. https://doi.org/10.1093/schbul/sbm047

Caplan, P. J. (1995). *They say you're crazy: How the world's most powerful psychiatrists decide who's normal.* Reading, MA: Addison-Wesley.

Cartwright, C., Gibson, K., Read, J., Cowan, O., & Dehar, T. (2016). Long-term antidepressant use: Patient perspectives of benefits and adverse effects. *Patient Preference and Adherence, 10*, 1401–1407.

Chung, D., Ryan, C., Hadzi-Pavlovic, D., Singh, S., Stanton, C., & Large, M. (2017). Suicide rates after discharge from psychiatric facilities: A systematic review and meta-analysis. *JAMA Psychiatry, 74*(7), 694–702. https://doi.org/10.1001/jamapsychiatry.2017.1044

Cohen, O. (2005). How do we recover? An analysis of psychiatric survivor oral histories. *Journal of Humanistic Psychology, 45*(3), 333–354.

Corin, E., Thara, R., & Padmavati, R. (2004). Living through the staggering world: The play of signifiers in early psychosis in South India. In J. H. Jenkins & R. J. Barrett (Eds.), *Schizophrenia, culture and subjectivity: The edge of experience.* Cambridge: Cambridge University Press.

Deacon, B. J. (2013). The biomedical model of mental disorder: A critical analysis of its validity, utility, and effects on psychotherapy research. *Clinical Psychology Review, 33*, 846–861.

Dell, P. F. (1998). Axis II pathology in outpatients with dissociative identity disorder. *Journal of Nervous and Mental Disorders, 186*, 352–356.

Dillon, J. (2013, March). Just saying it as it is: Names matter; Language matters; Truth matters. *Clinical Psychology Forum No. 243*: British Psychological Society.

Ellason, J. W., Ross, C. A., & Fuchs, D. L. (1996). Lifetime axis I and II comorbidity and childhood trauma history in dissociative identity disorder. *Psychiatry, 59*, 255–266.

Fenton, W. S., Mosher, L., Herrell, J. M., & Blyler, C. R. (1998). Randomized trial of general hospital and residential alternative care for patients with severe and persistent mental illness. *American Journal of Psychiatry, 155,* 516–522.

Fleischhacker, W. W., Kane, J. M., Geier, J., Karayal, O., Kolluri, S., Eng, S. M., … Strom, B. L. (2014). Completed and attempted suicides among 18,154 subjects with schizophrenia included in a large simple trial. *Journal of Clinical Psychiatry, 75*(3), e184–e190. https://doi.org/10.4088/JCP.13m08563

Gibson, S., Brand, S. L., Burt, S., Boden, Z. V., & Benson, O. (2013). Understanding treatment non-adherence in schizophrenia and bipolar disorder: A survey of what service users do and why. *BMC Psychiatry, 13*(1), 153.

Goldberg, D. (2011). The heterogeneity of "major depression". *World Psychiatry, 10*(3), 226–228.

Gotzsche, P. C. (2015). *Deadly psychiatry and organised denial.* Denmark: People's Press.

Greenfield, T. K., Stoneking, B. C., Humphreys, K., Sundby, E., & Bond, J. (2008). A randomized trial of a mental health consumer-managed alternative to civil commitment for acute psychiatric crisis. *American Journal of Community Psychology, 42,* 135–144.

Halpin, E., Kugathasan, V., Hulbert, C., Alvarez-Jimenez, M., & Bendall, S. (2016). Case formulation in young people with post-traumatic stress disorder and first-episode psychosis. *Journal of Clinical Medicine, 5*(11), 106. https://doi.org/10.3390/jcm5110106

Harrow, M., & Jobe, T. H. (2007). Factors involved in outcome and recovery in schizophrenia patients not on antipsychotic medications: A 15-year multifollow-up study. *The Journal of Nervous and Mental Disease, 195*(5), 406–414.

Harrow, M., Jobe, T. H., & Faull, R. N. (2012). Do all schizophrenia patients need antipsychotic treatment continuously throughout their lifetime? A 20-year longitudinal study. *Psychological Medicine, 42*(10), 2145–2155.

Healy, D. (2012). *Pharmageddon.* Los Angeles, CA: University of California Press.

Healy, D., Herxheimer, A., & Menkes, D. B. (2006). Antidepressants and violence: Problems at the interface of medicine and law. *Public Library of Science Medicine, 3*(9), e372.

Hjorthoj, C. R., Madsen, T., Agerbo, E., & Nordentoft, M. (2014). Risk of suicide according to level of psychiatric treatment: A nationwide nested case-control study. *Social Psychiatry and Psychiatric Epidemiology, 49,* 1357–1365.

Hofer, F. X., Habermeyer, E., Mokros, A., Lau, S., & Gairing, S. K. (2015). The impact of legal coercion on the therapeutic relationship in adult schizophrenic patients. *PLoS ONE, 10*(4), e0124043. https://doi.org/10.1371/journal.pone.0124043

Huber, C. G., Schneeberger, A. R., Kowalinski, E., Frohlich, D., von Felten, S., Walter, M., … Lang, U. E. (2016). Suicide risk and absconding in psychiatric hospitals with and without open door policies: A 15-year observational study. *Lancet Psychiatry, 3*(9), 842–849.

Human Rights Council. (2009, December). Thematic study by the Office of the United Nations High Commissioner for Human Rights on the structure and role of national mechanisms for the implementation and monitoring of the Convention on the Rights of Persons with Disabilities (A-HRC-13-29). *Annual report of the United Nations High Commissioner for Human Rights and reports of the Office of the High Commissioner and the Secretary-General.* Retrieved from http://www.ohchr.org/EN/Issues/Disability/Pages/ThematicStudies.aspx

Karon, B. P. (2000). *Effective psychoanalytic therapy of schizophrenia and other severe disorders.* Washington, DC: American Psychological Association.

Kisely, S. R., Campbell, L., & Preston, N. J. (2011). Compulsory community and involuntary outpatient treatment for people with severe mental disorders. *Cochrane Database of Systematic Reviews.* https://doi.org/10.1002/14651858. CD004408.pub3

Large, M., & Ryan, C. J. (2014). Disturbing findings about the risk of suicide and psychiatric hospitals. *Journal of Social Psychiatry and Psychiatric Epidemiology, 40*(9), 1353–1355.

Lloyd-Evans, B., Slade, M., Jagielska, D., & Johnson, S. (2009). Residential alternatives to acute psychiatric hospital admission: Systematic review. *British Journal of Psychiatry, 195,* 109–117.

Lucire, Y. (2016). Pharmacological iatrogenesis: Substance/medication-induced disorders that masquerade as mental illness. *Epidemiology, 6*(1). https://doi.org/10.4172/2161-1165.1000217

McHugh, R. K., Whitton, S. W., Peckham, A. D., Welge, J. A., & Otto, M. W. (2013). Patient preference for psychological vs. pharmacologic treatment of psychiatric disorders: A meta-analytic review. *Journal of Clinical Psychiatry, 74*(6), 595–602.

McWade, B. (2016). Recovery-as-policy as a form of neoliberal state making. *Intersectionalities: A Global Journal of Social Work Analysis, Research, Polity, and Practice, 5*(3), 62–81.

Mead, S., & Copeland, M. E. (2000). What recovery means to us: Consumers' perspectives. *Community Mental Health Journal, 36*(3), 315–328.

Mendez, J. E. (2013, March). Special Rapporteur on Torture and Other Cruel, Inhuman or Degrading Treatment or Punishment. 22nd session of the Human Rights Council, Agenda Item 3, Geneva.

Metzl, J. M. (2010). *The protest psychosis: How schizophrenia became a black disease.* Boston, MA: Beacon Press.

Moilanen, J., Haapea, M., Jaaskelainen, E., Veijola, J., Isohanni, M., Koponen, H., & Miettunen, J. (2016). Long-term antipsychotic use and its association with outcomes in schizophrenia – the Northern Finland Birth Cohort 1966. *European Psychiatry, 36,* 7–14.

Moncrieff, J., Cohen, D., & Porter, S. (2013). The psychoactive effects of psychiatric medication: The elephant in the room. *Journal of Psychoactive Drugs, 45*(5), 409–415. https://doi.org/10.1080/02791072.2013.845328

Moore, T. J., & Furberg, C. D. (2017). The harms of antipsychotic drugs: Evidence from key studies. *Drug Safety, 40*(1), 3–14.

Mueser, K. T., Lu, W., Rosenberge, S. D., & Wolfe, R. (2010). The trauma of psychosis: Posttraumatic stress disorder and recent onset psychosis. *Schizophrenia Research, 116*, 217–227.

Murphy, R., McGuinness, D., Bainbridge, E., Brosnan, L., Felzmann, H., Keys, M., ... Higgins, A. (2017). Service users' experiences of involuntary hospital admission under the Mental Health Act 2001 in the Republic of Ireland. *Psychiatric Services, 68*(11), 1127–1135.

Murray, R. M., Quattrone, D., Natesan, S., Van Os, J., Nordentoft, M., Howes, O., ... Taylor, D. (2016). Should psychiatrists be more cautious about the long-term prophylactic use of antipsychotics? *The British Journal of Psychiatry, 209*(5), 361–365.

Newnes, C. (2016). *Inscription, diagnosis, deception and the mental health industry.* London: Palgrave Macmillan.

Ostrow, L., Jessell, L., Hurd, M., Darrow, S. M., & Cohen, D. (2017). Discontinuing psychiatric medications: A survey of long-term users. *Psychiatric Services, 68*(12), 1232–1238.

Read, J. (2004). The invention of 'schizophrenia'. In J. Read, L. Mosher, & R. P. Bentall (Eds.), *Models of Madness.* East Sussex: Brunner-Routledge.

Read, J., & Arnold, C. (2017). Is electroconvulsive therapy for depression more effective than placebo? A systematic review of studies since 2009. *Ethical Human Psychology and Psychiatry, 19*(1), 5–23.

Rowe, M. (2013). Alternatives to outpatient commitment. *Journal of the American Academy of Psychiatry and the Law, 41*(3), 332–336.

Schizophrenia Commission. (2012, November). The abandoned illness: A report by the Schizophrenia commission. Retrieved from https://www.rethink.org/media/514093/TSC_main_report_14_nov.pdf

Seikkula, J., Alakare, B., & Aaltonen, J. (2011). The comprehensive open-dialogue approach in Western Lapland: II. Long-term stability of acute psychosis outcomes in advanced community care. *Psychosis, 3*, 192–204.

Skodol, A. E., Gunderson, J. G., Pfohl, B., Widiger, T. A., Livesley, W. J., & Siever, L. J. (2002). The borderline diagnosis I: Psychopathology, comorbidity, and personality structure. *Biological Psychiatry, 51*(12), 936–950.

Sledge, W. H., Tebes, J., Rakfeldt, J., Davidson, L., Lyons, L., & Druss, B. G. (1996). Day hospital/crisis respite care versus inpatient care, Part 1: Clinical outcomes. *American Journal of Psychiatry, 153*, 1065–1073.

Steadman, H., Gounis, K., Dennis, D., Hopper, K., Roche, B., Swartz, M., & Robbins, P. (2001). Assessing the New York city involuntary outpatient commitment pilot program. *Psychiatric Services, 52*(3), 330–336.

Tandon, R. (2014). Schizophrenia and other psychotic disorders in Diagnostic and Statistical Manual of Mental Disorders (DSM)-5: Clinical implications of revisions from DSM-IV. *Indian Journal of Psychological Medicine, 36*(3), 223–225. https://doi.org/10.4103/0253-7176.135365

The Lancet Psychiatry. (2017). Psychiatry unlocked. *The Lancet Psychiatry, 4*(4), 261. https://doi.org/10.1016/s2215-0366(17)30081-0

Thomas, P., & Longden, E. (2013). Madness, childhood adversity and narrative psychiatry: Caring and the moral imagination. *Medical Humanities, 39*(2), 119–125.

van Os, J. (2016). "Schizophrenia" does not exist. *BMJ, 352.* https://doi.org/10.1136/bmj.i375

Wardenaar, K. J., & de Jonge, P. (2013). Diagnostic heterogeneity in psychiatry: Towards an empirical solution. *BMC Medicine, 11*(1), 201. https://doi.org/10.1186/1741-7015-11-201

Whitaker, R. (2010). *Anatomy of an epidemic: Magic bullets, psychiatric drugs and the astonishing rise of mental illness.* New York, NY: Broadway Paperbacks.

Widiger, T. A., & Spitzer, R. L. (1991). Sex bias in the diagnosis of personality disorders: Conceptual and methodological issues. *Clinical Psychology Review, 11*(1), 1–22.

Wunderink, L., Nieboer, R. M., Wiersma, D., Sytema, S., & Nienhuis, F. J. (2013). Recovery in remitted first-episode psychosis at 7 years of follow-up of an early dose reduction/discontinuation or maintenance treatment strategy: Long-term follow-up of a 2-year randomized clinical trial. *JAMA Psychiatry, 70*(9), 913–920. https://doi.org/10.1001/jamapsychiatry.2013.19

CHAPTER 9

Recommendations and Moving Beyond
the System

> I think that one of the biggest problems with mental health [professionals]
> is that they really, really don't hear the mental health person. P10

In general, there are a myriad of different aspects of mental health treatment that may be helpful and/or harmful. Conversely, many individuals
may find their greatest healing once they are no longer in the mental
health system. There are clear implications of how the system and individual professionals may increase opportunities for healing for those seeking help. For instance, understanding the importance of taking a
client-centered, relational approach to working with individuals in emotional distress, appreciating the value of one's sense of agency and empowerment, realizing the sometimes inconsequential role that professionals
may play in some individuals' processes of recovery, and recognizing the
harms resultant from the current mental health paradigm are all major
recommendations for the field as a whole. In addition, it may be imperative that mental health professionals acknowledge that people's subjective
experiences are real, even if not always real to others, and to understand
the role of denial and shame from society as well as people seeking help.

Further, what is important to doctors and researchers may not be what
is essential to those whom they are purportedly helping. Recovery for
most is about contextualizing experiences within one's life narrative, making meaning, gaining hope, empowerment, learning to lead a healthy lifestyle, developing healthy relationships with self and other, and taking

© The Author(s) 2018   201
N. Hunter, *Trauma and Madness in Mental Health Services*,
https://doi.org/10.1007/978-3-319-91752-8_9

responsibility for one's own wellness, rather than "symptom reduction". There also is a need for services, overall, to become more trauma-informed, have a greater inclusion of people with lived experience in research and program development, and to gain an appreciation for lifestyle factors and peer support in the recovery process.

Taking a trauma-informed, client-led, non-medicalized perspective of the healing process may be one of the first steps that mental health professionals can take to improve services and outcomes. The lack of trauma-informed care often results in experiences where service users feel disrespected, intimidated, and re-traumatized, which obviously undermines their efforts to heal. More commonly, however, are the harms that result from a lack of knowledge or awareness of the ways in which standard practices can affect people who have experienced trauma. For instance, hospital wards may not always consider how particular customs, such as mixing genders on hospital wards, can be highly triggering and anxiety-inducing. Even worse, isolation in seclusion rooms and/or physical and chemical restraint can be directly traumatizing. Such practices may leave victims feeling fearful and suspicious yet further pathologized for an increased severity of "symptoms".

Simultaneously, however, people want to have care and precaution taken regarding their trauma histories, and also want to be respected for the strength, wisdom, and knowledge that they have to survive the experiences they suffered. It is also important, as part of a trauma-informed versus disease-based approach, for professionals to cease imparting defeatist prognoses and assumptions in favor of having a belief that all individuals have the possibility for recovery and a purposeful life. There needs to be a move away from a deficit-focused framework and consideration of the adaptive nature of the phenomena of concern (Ellis, Bianchi, Griskevicius, & Frankenhuis, 2017). This includes contextualizing experiences and attempting to understand phenomena that professionals may not have ever had themselves. For example, depression and anxiety are phenomena that professionals (and society) have an easier time empathizing with and understanding because they are common. On the other hand, with phenomena such as having dissociated parts, amnesia, altered states of consciousness, strange beliefs, voices, or other atypical experiences, people sometimes stop understanding and stop empathizing. Hope, validation, believing in a person, and trying to understand another's subjective experience can go a long way toward helping people heal and grow. Recovery rarely happens without these factors.

Believe in What You Do Not Understand

Believing your client is really important. P3

   She's the first person to believe ... and she got the father to admit to over a decade of abuse. And ... and ... that changed everything. She was the first person to believe ... [There was] no one in the mental health industry who took it seriously, or acted within the parameters of what I feel is acceptable behavior for a mental health professional. P12

   It's really helpful if someone just listens and says "I believe you. I believe you and the stories and sometimes things are more symbolic than others." P13

It was common for participants to have had their physical and emotional concerns dismissed, minimized, denied, and/or judged by professionals and society alike. Denial regarding one's level of distress or current dysfunction is particularly problematic for individuals who end up with a label of BPD or DID. This is partly due to their tendency to both exaggerate certain experiences as a result of chronic invalidation and also to react with numbness and dissociation of internal distress. It also is due to the prejudice and assumptions inherent in these diagnostic categories. Individuals with a diagnosis of DID are especially likely to be told that their experiences are not real due to the ideological belief that multiple self-parts are either a representation of malingering or a result of bad therapy (e.g., Piper, 1994; Piper & Merskey, 2005). Mental health and medical professionals are often experienced by service users as being dismissive of such individuals' expressions of pain and suffering, and being told they are "fine" even when they subjectively are terrified, hearing voices, confused, disoriented, disorganized, and/or suicidal (e.g., Sulzer, 2015).

   Additionally, it is also common for trauma survivors to engage in their own processes of denial and minimization (e.g., Goldsmith, Barlow, & Freyd, 2004), all of which can increase a sense of shame and worthlessness. Many trauma survivors have problems with memory or losing time, and so they cannot always report accurately on various experiences or, obviously, on what they have forgotten. On the other hand, denial, minimization, avoidance, and isolation are not always negative and may serve a purpose for some. These defenses may help individuals to function in the short-term, even if the result is feeling depressed, vulnerable to breakdown, and/or alone in the long run. Avoidance and isolation may also be responses to the intense shame and internalized prejudice that service users experience regarding both having a trauma history as well as emotional difficulties in a society that rejects extreme emotional distress.

It is essential that professionals take measures to ensure that they are not reinforcing these patterns and contributing to increased distress as a result.

Because denial, minimization, shame, stigma, and avoidance are so common for trauma survivors, as well as external figures in their lives, it is important for service users to have their experiences taken seriously, to not be judged, and not to be rejected for being difficult to understand or relate to. Instead of ignoring and trying to get rid of experiences such as voices, strange beliefs, or dissociated parts, these phenomena need to be directly worked with and explored. Suppressing these phenomena, as with any emotional experience, is ineffective, at best. For sure, it is recognized that direct work with things like dissociated parts or voices may result in temporarily increased dissociation and/or dysfunction, but it is, at times, necessary to meet people where they are at and work within, as opposed to against, their defensive system (Harper, 2011). These phenomena exist whether professionals or others ignore and suppress them or not.

People who have experienced chronic stress and adversity during childhood tend to have significant problems with memory, emotional numbness, and anxiety. Intense or anxiety-inducing behaviors on the part of service users, retraction of disclosures of abuse, spontaneous switches in mood or behavior, unpredictability, child-like mannerisms and speech, confusion about memories, and expression of emotions or experiences in a wooden or flat manner are also common for traumatized individuals. Unfortunately, this tends to result in professionals, family members, friends, and others accusing such individuals of attention-seeking, manipulating, lying, or being outright delusional. The believability of people is often questioned, particularly due to the indifferent attitude with which some individuals may react to such phenomena as seizures, flashbacks, or panic attacks (e.g., Foote, 1999). Yet, when one takes the time to contextualize a person's distress, understand the defensive nature of these problems, and to empathize with, rather than judge, these experiences, it becomes clear that few people are making up their histories, nor are they maliciously manipulating or lying (Goodman et al., 1999; Hegeman, 2009; Howell, 2005; Linehan, 1993).

For individuals who have experienced significant oppression, stress, and/or abuse within the family, secrecy, conflicting and unconvincing narratives, and retractions of abuse have long been acknowledged by clinicians as common (e.g., Summit, 1983). Memories for sexual abuse, specifically, tend to be dim, vague, and disavowed (Herman, 1992; Stern, 1996), further contributing to disbelief. In fact, severely dissociative individuals often have little to no memory for much of their trauma, and these memories may, instead, be experienced as unrecognizable intrusive visual images, symbolic acting out, metaphorical narratives, recurring nightmares, belonging to disowned parts of the self, and/or inexplicable somatic sensations (Davies, 1996; Howell, 2011; Van der Kolk, 1994). The conflicting, confusing, and bizarre displays of mysterious experiences only further lead to doubt and disbelief, and the feeling of the professional or others having been manipulated.

The importance of validation and believing service users does not necessarily equate with collusion or literal belief in the entirety of the person's subjective reality; rather, it is understanding the unique ways in which each individual may express his or her pain (i.e., metaphorical or symbolic belief systems, altered personality states, enactments, etc.) as well as validating the emotional experience and giving the person the benefit of the doubt that assertions of abuse are based in reality. Certainly, memories can be fallible (Koriat, Goldsmith, & Pansky, 2000) and certain practices can, indeed, lead to distorted memories (Scoboria, Mazzoni, Kirsch, & Milling, 2002), but this is not to discount that people have also experienced horrible acts of brutality and cruelty.

It also must be acknowledged and understood that people do sometimes forget/suppress/dissociate certain memories only to recall them later in life. There is a large body of research documenting cases of forgotten and then recalled abuse, sexual and physical assault, and neglect wherein such incidents were objectively verified as accurate (Feldman-Summers & Pope, 1994; Herman & Harvey, 1997; Krell, 1993; Scheflin & Brown, 1996; Widom & Shepard, 1996; Williams, 1995). Additionally, having periods of being completely unable to recall traumatic events only to later recall them appears to be common in traumatized populations, including war veterans and Holocaust survivors (Albach, Moormann, & Bermond, 1996; Wilsnack, Wonderlich, Kristjanson, Vogeltanz-Holm, & Wilsnack, 2002), and is associated with higher levels of posttraumatic distress (Elliott & Briere, 1995).

On the other hand, there are also many who have not had incidents of sexual or violent abuse occur in their lives and have either developed such a belief as a concrete metaphorical representation of more covert emotional abuse and/or have been led to believe otherwise by the seemingly well-intentioned practices of clinicians, friends, society, and oneself alike. Though fully formed "false memories" of traumatic events are thought by some to be rare (Stern, 1996), false beliefs do occur and can have detrimental consequences, including suicidal behaviors and attempts (e.g., Fetkewicz, Sharma, & Merskey, 2000). This is why it important to not insist on focusing on memory recall or repeated reliving of previous trauma, as narratives can and do become distorted. At the same time, one should always be given the benefit of the doubt that their memories are real and valid.

It may be more important for individuals to feel validated emotionally and learn to trust their own sense of reality without professionals suggesting what may or may not have happened. The best way that professionals can provide individuals with validation, acknowledgment, and a sense of safety while still challenging defenses is to have a non-judgmental space to discuss difficult subjects in the format of an open dialogue within a trusting relationship. The goal for many is to learn to trust oneself, to learn to tolerate not knowing, and to acknowledge and accept emotions as meaningful reactions to life events without needing to "recover memories" to do so. While service users need to be believed, it is also important that individuals, including professionals, need to be able to tolerate ambiguity and uncertainty. Insisting that service users present themselves and articulate their pain in a way that professionals understand is not only unempathic, it is also invalidating and harmful. At the end of the day, as stated by P8: "It's [about] whether you're being appropriate or not, and if you're not hurting anyone, who gives a shit?"

NOTHING ABOUT US WITHOUT US

Much of the professional literature is based on an outside perspective that rarely includes the expertise of those individuals who have actually experienced the phenomena of evaluation or study. At the same time, a major goal of researchers who actually have lived experience tends to be to challenge accepted knowledge and expand perspectives beyond the status quo (e.g., Ingram, 2016). Berta Britz (2017), a powerful advocate within the Hearing Voices Movement, stands with many other advocates (Smith, 2016; Sweeney, 2016) in calling for providers and researchers to include service users and to truly be open to hearing and connecting with persons under study in an inclusive manner focused on mutual learning. Any venture that has a goal of increasing understanding, developing knowledge, and discovering new possibilities requires openness to multiple viewpoints, disparate voices, and an appreciation for all stakeholders involved. Thus far, individuals with lived experience of mental health services have traditionally been ignored and actively left out of the equation. This must change.

For a doctor to insinuate what is best for a person with lived experiences that said doctor has never had is akin to a man telling a woman what she needs to be sexually satisfied, happy, or fulfilled in work. Of course, in the not-so-distant past this was exactly how most cultures operated. Just as times have changed for women, so too must they change for people who experience emotional distress and/or enter into mental health services. These experts-by-experience offer unique perspectives and should be included as equal participants at all levels of research and design and implementation of intervention services. The World Health Organization (2010) has described the need for promoting the inclusion of people with lived experience as a human rights agenda.

A collaborative approach is more likely to honor individual, subjective considerations of what constitutes recovery, what is most important for functional and purposeful living, and how best to achieve these goals. These subjective experiences tend to include an understanding of oppression, discrimination, severe abuse, marginalization, loss and helplessness to which few doctors can relate on an experiential level. Further, those who have found ways to heal and move through their difficulties can provide practical guidance for others, which often is much broader and meaningful than "symptom management".

For many services users across all areas of mental health, recovery and what it takes to achieve it means something very different than that of the professional (Bellack, 2006; Neale et al., 2015; Ng et al., 2008). Participants expressed goals of feeling human, empowerment, making meaningful contributions to society, building relationships, decreasing overall distress, feeling safe, and accepting all parts of their selves in all of their various manifestations. Consistent with this, throughout the literature, recovery for service users is often about coping with their specific difficulties in an empowering manner that allows them to lead a functional, productive, and satisfying life with a healthy support network and a respectful acceptance of oneself (Cohen, 2005; Dillon & May, 2002; Leamy, Bird, Le Boutillier, Williams, & Slade, 2011; Mead & Copeland, 2000; Thornhill, Clare, & May, 2004). What service users generally want is to increase their quality of life and simply feel better about themselves (Byrne & Morrison, 2014), which looks different for any given individual.

Perhaps most importantly, professionals need to believe that recovery is even possible in the first place. People can and do recover. And, recovery is not necessarily about the permanent absence of "symptoms" or distressing emotions/behavior. Rather, finding meaning, purpose, employment, and having a high quality of life is possible for most, regardless of what unique psychic phenomena one may or may not experience. This should be considered the norm without shaming those who may, nonetheless, struggle intensely throughout life. If this fact is accepted, then the idea that such individuals might have important insights to offer the professional realm is clearly evident.

BEYOND THE SYSTEM

My friends have really been more helpful than anything else ... It's so helpful to know that when I'm having a hard time, I have people in my life who genuinely care what's going on. P1

Ya know, a lot of stuff doesn't happen in therapy. P3

What I discovered was that massive amounts of healing don't happen in therapy and it certainly doesn't happen in isolation. It happens in engaging in life. P5

Many people who recover from histories of chronic trauma, adversity, and oppression find much of their healing outside of formal services, or even in spite of these services. The single most important factor in the healing process is forming safe and healthy relationships, which may or may not be in the form of a mental health professional. Engaging in more healthy lifestyles and finding peer support, formally or not, can provide the platform for long-lasting change. This can be a part of a formal therapeutic process or be entirely separate from any professional service at all. Professional services are an important, but not necessary, part of the equation. People have been healing and overcoming emotional pain since the beginning of time with and without the need for doctors.

Lifestyle Changes

Certain activities are just calming and therapeutic. I guess just, like, walking, meditation type of things. P7

Attending to outside lifestyle factors from stage one of therapy or any recovery process is imperative. For many, what happens outside of therapy, such as speaking with friends, peers, family, exercise, and/or engaging in self-help programs or activities, can be more helpful, safer, and more effective than much of what is experienced with any professional. Many clinicians are biased to perceive changes in their patients as due to the therapy process (Lilienfeld, Ritschel, Lynn, Cautin, & Latzman, 2014) or as more beneficial than they are (Hoffman & Del Mar, 2017). Yet, when looking at the overall statistics, psychotherapy tends to only have a nominally statistically significant effect with little convincing evidence that it is as powerful as society is generally led to believe (Cristea et al., 2017; Dragioti, Karathanos, Gerdle, & Evangelou, 2017). Recovery narratives often tend to attribute changes largely to factors such as cultural and personal experiences outside of professional help (e.g., Judge, Estroff, Perkins, & Penn, 2008).

Having supportive family and friends in one's life is central to the recovery process. In fact, phenomena such as voices or dissociated self-parts tend to be reflective of social and familial relationships (Vilhauer, 2016), suggesting that there may be a reciprocal effect of working on both relationship with self and self-parts as well as relationships in the social world. Learning to assert oneself and establishing appropriate boundaries that can help a person feel safe and empowered is a primary goal for many. When people experience trusting relationships and are engaged in purposeful activities, they report being able to learn and grow in their own unique ways that leads to improved quality of life (Bertram & McDonald, 2015). Even with engagement in therapy, these relationships are paramount. Participants believed that they would not have been able to survive or tolerate the therapeutic process if it had not been for people in their life who supported and believed in them.

This relationship building also includes building empathy for and helping others. For many, maintaining relationships with other individuals from hospital or peer support groups where they could equally rely upon and help these peers was empowering and boosted their self-worth. Helping others and volunteering for helping causes has been demonstrated to decrease the stress response, even at the biological and genetic level, for some (e.g., Poulin & Holman, 2013; Sneed & Cohen, 2013). It also helps to understand that one is not alone in suffering and can bring people out of a narrow victim role into one that is more human and whole.

In order for people to grow and recover from adversity, it is crucial that they focus on their whole selves and develop a sense of value and worth. This includes engaging in activities that provide a sense of empowerment and purpose. Finding meaning in life and discerning what past psychological and life experiences mean in the context of a greater existential purpose can be profoundly healing. This can be explored and discovered through attending to spirituality, whether it be formal religion or simply focusing on the existential in relationship and/or in therapy. Most people who have experienced chronic adversity and/or oppression tend to have an over-whelming sense of injustice, loss of meaning in life, and existential pain that can only be processed or understood through a spiritual lens. In this vein, "trauma work" is not so much about reliving the past, but coming to understand how and why such suffering exists, making sense of it, and sharing in common existential perspectives with others.

Some spiritual practices, outside of formal religion, that can be particu-larly helpful, especially in helping to calm and ground a person when feel-ing anxious, or over- or under-aroused, are activities such as yoga, meditation, and mindfulness practices. Yoga (Prathikanti et al., 2017) and mediation/mindfulness (Eisendrath et al., 2008; Geschwind, Peeters, Drukker, van Os, & Wichers, 2011) have been shown to reduce depres-sion and increase a sense of self-esteem and self-efficacy, to help trauma-tized youth in juvenile justice settings (see Epstein & Gonzalez, 2017 for a review), to reduce overall posttraumatic distress at least as well as formal psychotherapy and/or psychotropic drugs (van der Kolk et al., 2014), and, for those who maintain a consistent yoga practice, a loss of the diag-nosis of PTSD (Rhodes, Spinazzola, & van der Kolk, 2016). Exercise, in general, has been shown to decrease emotional distress, including those experiences often labeled as psychotic, and improves confidence, global functioning, memory, attention, social cognition, and a sense of achieve-ment (Blumenthal et al., 1999; Firth et al., 2016, 2017; Hillman, Erickson, & Kramer, 2008; Kim et al., 2014; Ten Brinke et al., 2014).

Being in touch with nature also has powerful effects on mental well-being (e.g., Bratman, Hamilton, Hahn, Daily, & Gross, 2015). A study by de Vries et al. (2016) found evidence to support the idea that individuals who live near trees, plants, and water tend to have better mental and phys-ical health, overall. Sometimes taking a walk and being able to just see plants or breathe clean air is enough to feel grounded and connected. In sum, taking care of the body and soul, forming healthy relationships, and connecting with nature all can be incredibly powerful in the healing process and, for some, may be enough to work through and overcome adverse experiences.

Peer Support

Peer support … was helpful … I thought that they were the only ones that could understand what I was even talking about. P2

Healing requires you helping someone and someone helping you. P4

Peer support is increasingly being recognized as an important component in healing, whether in addition to or independent of more formal mental health treatment. Organized peer support has its roots largely in the consumer movement of the 1970s, wherein service users began protesting standard mental health interventions and finding ways to help themselves and each other. Engaging in peer support, whether in person or online, can help a person feel included, understood, and supported, rather than pathologized, judged, and marginalized, as often happens within the mental health system. It also helps individuals understand that they are not the only ones to suffer in life, and increases empathy for those who have and do suffer in similar and different ways. Benefits not typically found in mental health services may also be found through support by those with lived experience (e.g., Repper & Carter, 2011), such as empowerment, meaning-making, and connection.

Peer support helps individuals across diagnostic categories to feel more empowered, hopeful, and capable (Davidson, Bellamy, Guy, & Miller, 2012; Mahlke et al., 2017). Greenfield, Stoneking, Humphreys, Sundby, and Bond (2008) found, in a randomized controlled trial, that individuals who were assisted in a peer-run respite center during crisis had increased improvement in distress, increased service satisfaction, and 33% less cost than those who were treated in a psychiatric hospital. Peer-run services appear to be better tolerated and less intrusive, as well as have little to no association with traumatization of individuals or increased suicides. Further, they may provide opportunities to form and improve interpersonal relationships (Davidson et al., 2012), which, as discussed previously, is central in the recovery process.

The Hearing Voices Network (HVN) is one example of peer support that has been progressively appreciated internationally as providing a new way of thinking about and working with atypical experiences, such as hearing voices. These groups have been widely studied and increasingly have empirical support for their use (e.g., Longden, Read, & Dillon, 2018). Hearing voices groups are run by and for individuals who hear voices and experience other atypical phenomena, such as having belief systems others may not understand. They are open to any and all individual frames for understanding these experiences, even medical model perspectives, support individual decisions pertaining to the use of psychiatric drugs, and are focused on finding meaning within one's experiences and learning ways to cope with trauma, psychic or spiritual pain, and voice-hearing. It operates on the premise that voices, and other extrasensory experiences, are metaphorical representations of conflicts most often related to trauma. Professional treatments based on this self-help network utilize a phase-based, trauma-informed, non-diagnostic approach that focuses on stabilization, working through internal conflicts and trauma, and recovery (Romme, Escher, Dillon, Corstens, & Morris, 2009). The goal is not to get rid of voices, or other anomalous experiences, but rather to understand the meaning behind their development, regain control and empowerment, and find compassion toward and cooperation between and with the voices or parts.

A recent review by Beavan, de Jager, and dos Santos (2017) demonstrated consistent evidence for how these groups result in increased self-confidence and self-esteem, an increased sense of empowerment, decreased isolation, and an increased sense of understanding of the voices. The emphasis on understanding voices and meaning-making is based on the research showing that the voices, themselves, are not the problem so much as problems with coping and negotiating with them and finding meaning in the experience (Baumeister, Sedgwick, Howes, & Peters, 2017; Corstens, Escher, & Romme, 2008; Longden, Corstens, Escher, & Romme, 2012; Payne, Allen, & Lavender, 2017; Powers, Kelley, & Corlett, 2016). As expressed by Longden et al. (2018), "it is intuitive that providing a safe, communal forum in which individuals assemble to share coping strategies, validate one another's stories, and exchange wisdom and insights, can reduce shame and isolation and expedite a greater sense of acceptance for an experience that is both distressing and highly stigmatized." Exploring experiences of voice-hearing, atypical beliefs, dissociated parts, and other phenomena generally suppressed by most mental health frameworks is paramount to better understanding the whole self, linking past experiences of trauma and adversity to current difficulties, meaning-making, decreased sense of defectiveness or otherness, and self-acceptance.

The Hearing Voices Network has become popular, but by no means is the only form of peer support. There are innumerable ways in which peer support may be offered, from the formal employment of peers in traditional services, less formal independent groups, or simply befriending someone who gets you and has been there. Online peer support, in particular, can provide a forum for a person to feel safe, and have a sense of confidentiality and control in when and how he or she communicates. Such forums may offer connection, individualized adaptation, education, shared experiences, and promotion of positive coping strategies (Coulson, Bullock, & Rodham, 2017). Peer support groups can also help some people to feel motivated and supported to engage more fully in therapy or other formal services. Additionally, helping others while in a peer role, or in any role, is inspiring, gives meaning to one's own painful experiences, and provides a sense of purpose and meaning, all of which are vital components to the recovery process.

Overall, increasing quality of life and finding a purpose in life is a vital goal of the healing process. Being able to enjoy life, having a purpose to live for, having hope and something that keeps people going are basic human needs. People who seek out mental health services are generally just wanting to live a functional life, with meaning and purpose, and to feel like a whole person that is not perceived as broken or ill. In other words, there is no "us" and "them"—we all, every human, just wants to lead a meaningful and content life wherein one's unique experiences and characteristics can be honored and appreciated without discrimination or oppression. A utopian dream, perhaps, but certainly such a dream can begin being realized by a field that ostensibly is designed to specifically provide a safe healing opportunity for society's most vulnerable.

REFERENCES

Albach, F., Moormann, P. P., & Bermond, B. (1996). Memory recovery of childhood sexual abuse. *Dissociation, 9*(4), 261–273.

Baumeister, D., Sedgwick, O., Howes, O., & Peters, E. (2017). Auditory verbal hallucinations and continuum models of psychosis: A systematic review of the healthy voice-hearer literature. *Clinical Psychology Review, 51*, 125–141.

Beavan, V., de Jager, A., & dos Santos, B. (2017). Do peer-support groups for voice-hearers work? A small scale study of Hearing Voices Network support groups in Australia. *Psychosis, 9*(1), 57–66.

Bellack, A. S. (2006). Scientific and consumer models of recovery in schizophrenia: Concordance, contrasts, and implications. *Schizophrenia Bulletin, 32*(3), 432–442.

Bertram, M., & McDonald, S. (2015). From surviving to thriving: How does that happen. *The Journal of Mental Health Training: Education and Practice, 10*(5), 337–348.

Blumenthal, J. A., Babyak, M. A., Moore, K. A., Craighead, W. E., Herman, S., Khatri, P., ... Krishnan, K. R. (1999). Effects of exercise training on older patients with major depression. *Archives of Internal Medicine, 159*(19), 2349–2356. https://doi.org/10.1001/archinte.159.19.2349

Bratman, G. N., Hamilton, J. P., Hahn, K. S., Daily, G. C., & Gross, J. J. (2015). Nature experience reduces rumination and subgenual prefrontal cortex activation. *PNAS, 112*(28), 8567–8572.

Britz, B. (2017). Listening and hearing: A voice hearer's invitation into relationship. *Frontiers in Psychology*. https://doi.org/10.3389/fpsyg.2017.00387

Byrne, R., & Morrison, A. P. (2014). Service users' priorities and preferences for treatment of psychosis: A user-led Delphi study. *Psychiatric Services, 65*, 1167–1169.

Cohen, O. (2005). How do we recover? An analysis of psychiatric survivor oral histories. *Journal of Humanistic Psychology, 45*(3), 333–354.

Corstens, D., Escher, S., & Romme, M. (2008). Accepting and working with voices: The Maastricht approach. In A. Moskowitz, I. Schafer, & M. J. Dorahy (Eds.), *Psychosis, trauma and dissociation: Emerging perspectives on severe psychopathology* (pp. 319–332). Chichester: Wiley-Blackwell.

Coulson, S. N., Bullock, E., & Rodham, K. (2017). Exploring the therapeutic affordances of self-harm online support communities: An online survey of members. *JMIR Mental Health, 4*(4), e44. https://doi.org/10.2196/mental.8084

Cristea, I. A., Gentili, C., Cotet, C. D., Palomba, D., Barbui, C., & Cuijpers, P. (2017). Efficacy of psychotherapies for borderline personality disorder: A systematic review and meta-analysis. *JAMA Psychiatry, 74*(4), 319–328.

Davidson, L., Bellamy, C., Guy, K., & Miller, R. (2012). Peer support among persons with severe mental illnesses: A review of evidence and experience. *World Psychiatry, 11*(2), 123–128.

Davies, J. M. (1996). Dissociation, repression and reality testing in the countertransference: The controversey over memory and false memory in the psychoanalytic treatment of adult survivors of childhood sexual abuse. *Psychoanalytic Dialogues, 6*(2), 189–218.

de Vries, S., ten Have, M., van Dorsselaer, S., van Wezep, M., Hermans, T., & de Graaf, R. (2016). Local availability of green and blue space and prevalence of common mental disorders in the Netherlands. *British Journal of Psychiatry Open, 2*(6), 366–372.

Dillon, J., & May, R. (2002). Reclaiming experience. *Clinical Psychology, 17*, 25–77.

Dragioti, E., Karathanos, V., Gerdle, B., & Evangelou, E. (2017). Does psychotherapy work? An umbrella review of meta-analyses of randomized controlled trials. [Review]. *Acta Psychiatrica Scandinavica, 136*(3), 236–246.

Eisendrath, S. J., Delucchi, K., Bitner, R., Fenimore, P., Smit, M., & McLane, M. (2008). Mindfulness-based cognitive therapy for treatment-resistant depression: A pilot study. *Psychotherapy and Psychosomatics, 77*(5), 319–320.

Elliott, D. M., & Briere, J. (1995). Posttraumatic stress associated with delayed recall of sexual abuse: A general population study. *Journal of Traumatic Stress, 8*(4), 629–647.

Ellis, B. J., Bianchi, J. M., Griskevicius, V., & Frankenhuis, W. E. (2017). Beyond risk and protective factors: An adaptation-based approach to resilience.

Perspectives on Psychological Science, 12(4), 561–587. https://doi.org/10.1177/1745691617693054

Epstein, R., & Gonzalez, T. (2017). Gender & trauma: Somatic interventions for girls in juvenile justice: Implications for policy and practice. Retrieved from http://www.law.georgetown.edu/academics/centers-institutes/poverty-inequality/upload/gender-and-trauma.pdf

Feldman-Summers, S., & Pope, K. S. (1994). The experiences of "forgetting" childhood abuse: A national survey of psychologists. *Journal of Consulting and Clinical Psychology, 62*(3), 636–639.

Fetkewicz, J., Sharma, V., & Merskey, H. (2000). A note on suicidal deterioration with recovery memory treatment. *Journal of Affective Disorders, 58*, 155–159.

Firth, J., Carney, R., Elliott, R., French, P., Parker, S., McIntyre, R. S., ... Yung, A. R. (2016). Exercise as an intervention for first-episode psychosis: A feasibility study. *Early Intervention in Psychiatry.* https://doi.org/10.1111/eip.12329

Firth, J., Stubbs, B., Rosenbaum, S., Vancampfort, D., Malchow, B., Schuch, F., ... Yung, A. R. (2017). Aerobic exercise improves cognitive functioning in people with schizophrenia: A systematic review and meta-analysis. *Schizophrenia Bulletin, 43*(3), 546–556.

Foote, B. (1999). Dissociative identity disorder and pseudo-hysteria. *American Journal of Psychotherapy, 53*(3), 320–343.

Geschwind, N., Peeters, F., Drukker, M., van Os, J., & Wichers, M. (2011). Mindfulness training increases momentary positive emotions and reward experiences in adults vulnerable to depression: A randomized controlled trial. *Journal of Consulting and Clinical Psychology, 79*(5), 618–628.

Goldsmith, R. E., Barlow, M. R., & Freyd, J. J. (2004). Knowing and not knowing about trauma: Implications for therapy. *Psychotherapy: Theory, Research, Practice, Training, 41*(4), 448–463.

Goodman, L., Thompson, K. M., Weinfurt, K., Corl, S., Acker, P., Mueser, K. T., & Rosenberg, S. D. (1999). Reliability of reports of violent victimization and posttraumatic stress disorder among men and women with serious mental illness. *Journal of Traumatic Stress, 12*(4), 587–599.

Greenfield, T. K., Stoneking, B. C., Humphreys, K., Sundby, E., & Bond, J. (2008). A randomized trial of a mental health consumer-managed alternative to civil commitment for acute psychiatric crisis. *American Journal of Community Psychology, 42*, 135–144.

Harper, S. (2011). An examination of structural dissociation of the personality and the implications for cognitive behavioural therapy. *The Cognitive Behaviour Therapist, 4*, 53–67.

Hegeman, E. (2009). One or many? Commentary on paper by Debra Rothschild. *Psychoanalytic Dialogues, 19*, 188–196.

Herman, J. (1992). *Trauma and recovery.* New York: Basic Books.

Herman, J., & Harvey, M. R. (1997). Adult memories of childhood trauma: A naturalistic clinical study. *Journal of Traumatic Stress, 10*(4), 557–571.

Hillman, C. H., Erickson, K. I., & Kramer, A. F. (2008). Be smart, exercise your heart: Exercise effects on brain and cognition. *Nature Reviews Neuroscience, 9*, 58–65.

Hoffman, T. C., & Del Mar, C. (2017). Clinicians' expectations of the benefits and harms of treatments, screenings, and tests: A systematic review. *JAMA Internal Medicine, 177*(3), 407–419.

Howell, E. (2005). *The dissociative mind.* London: Routledge.

Howell, E. (2011). *Understanding and treating dissociative identity disorder: A relational approach.* New York, NY: Taylor and Francis Group, LLC.

Ingram, R. A. (2016). Doing mad studies: Making (non)sense together. *Intersectionalities: A Global Journal of Social Work Analysis, Research, Polity, and Practice, 5*(3), 11–17.

Judge, A. M., Estroff, S. E., Perkins, D. O., & Penn, D. L. (2008). Recognizing and responding to early psychosis: A qualitative analysis of individual narratives. *Psychiatric Services, 59*(1), 96–99.

Kim, H. J., Song, B. K., So, B., Lee, O., Song, W., & Kim, Y. (2014). Increase of circulating BDNF levels and its relation to improvement of physical fitness following 12 weeks of combined exercise in chronic patients with schizophrenia: A pilot study. *Psychiatry Research, 220*(3), 792–796.

Koriat, A., Goldsmith, M., & Pansky, A. (2000). Toward a psychology of memory accuracy. *Annual Review of Psychology, 51*, 481–537.

Krell, R. (1993). Child survivors of the Holocaust: Strategies of adaptation. *The Canadian Journal of Psychiatry, 38*(6), 384–389.

Leamy, M., Bird, V., Le Boutillier, C., Williams, J., & Slade, M. (2011). Conceptual framework for personal recovery in mental health: Systematic review and narrative synthesis. *The British Journal of Psychiatry, 199*, 445–452.

Lilienfeld, S. O., Ritschel, L. A., Lynn, S. J., Cautin, R. L., & Latzman, R. D. (2014). Why ineffective psychotherapies appear to work: A taxonomy of causes of spurious therapeutic effectiveness. *Perspectives on Psychological Science, 9*(4), 355–387.

Linehan, M. M. (1993). *Cognitive behavioral treatment of borderline personality disorder.* New York, NY: The Guilford Press.

Longden, E., Corstens, D., Escher, S., & Romme, M. (2012). Voice hearing in a biographical context: A model for formulating the relationship between voices and life history. *Psychosis, 4*(3), 224–234.

Longden, E., Read, J., & Dillon, J. (2018). Assessing the impact and effectiveness of Hearing Voices Network self-help groups. *Community Mental Health Journal, 54*(2), 184–188.

Mahlke, C. I., Priebe, S., Heumann, K., Daubmann, A., Weqscheider, K., & Bock, T. (2017). Effectiveness of one-to-one peer support for patients with severe mental illness – A randomized controlled trial. *European Psychiatry, 42*, 103–110.

Mead, S., & Copeland, M. E. (2000). What recovery means to us: Consumers' perspectives. *Community Mental Health Journal, 36*(3), 315–328.

Neale, J., Tompkins, C., Wheeler, C., Finch, E., Marsden, J., Mitcheson, L., … Strang, J. (2015). "You're all going to hate the word 'recovery' by the end of this": Service users' views of measuring addiction recovery. *Drugs: Education, Prevention and Policy, 22*(1), 26–34. https://doi.org/10.3109/09687637.20 14.947564

Ng, R. M., Pearson, V., Lam, M., Law, C. W., Chiu, C. P., & Chen, E. Y. (2008). What does recovery from schizophrenia mean? Perceptions of long-term patients. *International Journal of Social Psychiatry, 54*(2), 118–130.

Payne, T., Allen, J., & Lavender, T. (2017). Hearing voices network groups: Experiences of eight voice hearers and the connection to group processes and recovery. *Psychosis, 9*(3), 205–215.

Piper, A., Jr. (1994). Treatment for multiple personality disorder: At what cost? *American Journal of Psychotherapy, 48*(3), 392–400.

Piper, A., Jr., & Merskey, H. (2005). Reply: The persistence of folly: A critical examination of dissociative identity disorder. *The Canadian Journal of Psychiatry, 50*(12), 814.

Poulin, M. J., & Holman, E. A. (2013). Helping hands, healthy body? Oxytocin receptor gene and prosocial behavior interact to buffer the association between stress and physical health. *Hormones and Behavior, 63*(3), 510–517. https://doi.org/10.1016/j.yhbeh.2013.01.004

Powers, A. R., III, Kelley, M. S., & Corlett, P. R. (2016). Varieties of voice-hearing: Psychics and the psychosis continuum. *Schizophrenia Bulletin, 43*(1), 84–98.

Prathikanti, S., Rivera, R., Cochran, A., Tungol, J. G., Fayazmanesh, N., & Weinmann, E. (2017). Treating major depression with yoga: A prospective, randomized, controlled pilot trial. *PLoS ONE, 12*(3), e0173869.

Repper, J., & Carter, T. (2011). A review of the literature on peer support in mental health services. *Journal of Mental Health, 20*(4), 392–411.

Rhodes, A., Spinazzola, J., & van der Kolk, B. A. (2016). Yoga for adult women with chronic PTSD: A long-term follow-up study. *The Journal of Alternative and Complementary Medicine, 22*(3), 189–196.

Romme, M., Escher, S., Dillon, J., Corstens, D., & Morris, M. (Eds.). (2009). *Living with voices: 50 stories of recovery*. Herefordshire: PCCS Books Ltd.

Scheflin, A. W., & Brown, D. (1996). Repressed memory of dissociative amnesia: What the science says. *Journal of Psychiatry & Law, 24*(2), 143–188.

Scoboria, A., Mazzoni, G., Kirsch, I., & Milling, L. S. (2002). Immediate and persisting effects of misleading questions and hypnosis on memory reports. *Journal of Experimental Psychology, 8*, 26–32.

Smith, C. B. R. (2016). "About nothing without us": A comparative analysis of autonomous organizing among people who use drugs and psychiatrized groups in Canada. *Intersectionalities: A Global Journal of Social Work Analysis, Research, Polity, and Practice, 5*(3), 82–109.

Sneed, R. S., & Cohen, S. (2013). A prospective study of volunteerism and hypertension risk in older adults. *Psychology and Aging, 28*(2), 578–586. https://doi.org/10.1037/a0032718

Stern, D. B. (1996). Dissociation and constructivism: Commentary on papers by Davies and Harris. *Psychoanalytic Dialogues, 6*(2), 251–266.

Sulzer, S. H. (2015). Does "difficult patient" status contribute to de facto demedicalization? The case of borderline personality disorder. *Social Science & Medicine, 142*, 82–89. https://doi.org/10.1016/j.socscimed.2015.08.008

Summit, R. C. (1983). The child abuse accommodation syndrome. *Child Abuse & Neglect, 7*, 177–193.

Sweeney, A. (2016). Why mad studies needs survivor research and survivor research needs mad studies. *Intersectionalities: A Global Journal of Social Work Analysis, Research, Polity, and Practice, 5*(3), 36–61.

Ten Brinke, L. F., Bolandzadeh, N., Nagamatsu, L. S., Hsu, C. L., Davis, J. C., Miran-Khan, K., & Liu-Ambrose, T. (2014). Aerobic exercise increases hippocampal volume in older women with probable mild cognitive impairment: A 6-month randomised controlled trial. *British Journal of Sports Medicine, 49*(4), 248–254.

Thornhill, H., Clare, L., & May, R. (2004). Escape, enlightenment and endurance: Narratives of recovery from psychosis. *Anthropology & Medicine, 11*(2), 181–199.

Van der Kolk, B. A. (1994). The body keeps the score: Memory and the evolving psychobiology of posttraumatic stress. *Harvard Review of Psychiatry, 1*, 253–265.

van der Kolk, B. A., Stone, L., West, J., Rhodes, A., Emerson, D., Suvak, M., & Spinazzola, J. (2014). Yoga as an adjunctive treatment for posttraumatic stress disorder: A randomized controlled trial. *Journal of Clinical Psychiatry, 75*(6), e559–e565.

Vilhauer, R. P. (2016). Stigma and need for care in individuals who hear voices. *International Journal of Social Psychiatry, 63*(1), 5–13. https://doi.org/10.1177/0020764016675888

Widom, C. S., & Shepard, R. L. (1996). Accuracy of adult recollections of childhood victimization. Part 1. Childhood physical abuse. *Psychological Assessment, 8*(4), 412–421.

Williams, L. M. (1995). Recovered memories of abuse in women with documented child sexual victimization histories. *Journal of Traumatic Stress, 8*(4), 649–673.

Wilsnack, S. C., Wonderlich, S. A., Kristjanson, A. F., Vogeltanz-Holm, N. D., & Wilsnack, R. W. (2002). Self-reports of forgetting and remembering childhood sexual abuse in a nationally representative sample of US women. *Child Abuse & Neglect, 26,* 139–147.

World Health Organization. (2010). *User empowerment in mental health: A statement by the WHO regional office for Europe.* Copenhagen: World Health Organization.

CHAPTER 10

Resources and Helpful Tips

Some of the stuff, I guess, is not really directly involved with a therapist or psychiatrist, some of it's just on my own. Stuff that I have found that has been helpful or that has worked for me. P3

I got a lot of my ideas from, really, a lot of sources—philosophy, sociology, neuropsychiatry … I draw a lot more widely, and I've found it a lot more useful. P5

A big piece of it is also, not just what the therapist does, but it's also on you. P11

While there are many criticisms of standard mental health care presented throughout this book, the therapeutic process can, for many, be incredibly healing and helpful. At the same time, therapy is not for everyone, nor can everyone afford therapy or has insurance to cover the costs. The following provides suggested ways to find a therapist as well as resources for finding groups and supports outside of formal services. Of course, none of these is mutually exclusive; each person's journey is their own and it is unlikely that just one thing is going to be *the* answer. No matter how people put together a support network and build relationships, it is always important to find ways to care for the self. This chapter ends with tips on self-care and coping with some of the phenomena explored throughout this book. Note that nothing presented here is intended as medical advice; rather, these are ideas that may or may not be helpful for any given individual and as suggested by others who have

© The Author(s) 2018
N. Hunter, *Trauma and Madness in Mental Health Services*,
https://doi.org/10.1007/978-3-319-91752-8_10

found these things to be helpful for them. Hopefully, it helps provide some initial direction for people to discover their own unique path toward healing.

FINDING A HELPFUL THERAPIST

But I do have a therapist now who's really great. P1

When I did eventually get to see someone, I didn't realize there were trauma specialists, but there were. So I went to see my GP to get a referral. She was really lovely, managed it really well, sent me to the lady I'm now seeing. I've been seeing her for five years. So, yeah, things have been good since I've been seeing her. P8

Establishing a bond with the therapist that is based on mutual trust and respect [is important]. P12

Navigating the seemingly endless options of therapists in some geographical areas (and lack of options in others!) can feel overwhelming and impossible, at times, especially if already stressed and/or scared. Nonetheless, it is a task that is best not rushed or taken lightly when considering the central importance of the therapeutic relationship in the healing process. You should feel like you have chosen the person you are working with, not that you settled for or feel obligated to them in some way.

The process of finding a therapist may begin by being given referrals after a crisis situation, seeing someone a parent or other family member set up, or starting with a school-based counselor. These are not ideal situations, but sometimes great relationships can be born out of chance circumstances. Ideally, however, you will have the opportunity to choose for yourself, and that often begins by asking around for referrals or searching online. In this initial search, you want to find someone who is comfortable working with your particular issues, as you perceive and describe them, and whose biography (usually found online) resonates with you. Once you have an initial list, start by calling or emailing. You want to make sure they are taking on new clients, that scheduling is feasible, they are affordable and/or take your insurance, and are politely responsive. Personally, perhaps because I struggle, and always have, with telephone interactions and "selling" myself, I do not ascribe too much weight to these initial correspondences beyond determining logistics and general kindness. On the other hand, if you get a bad vibe, for whatever reason, then just move on to the next person on the list.

The first in-person interview, however, is much more indicative of who the clinician might be, how he or she behaves, and if the relationship might be a fruitful one. One should never feel like they are being disrespected, judged, looked down upon, or made to feel crazy. A therapeutic relationship is one in which a person needs to feel supported, understood, heard, valued, and safe. At the same time, the past can make it difficult to trust others, and one might perceive judgment, disrespect, and dismissiveness where there is none. Further, avoidance is a pretty common habit for many of us, and it might be worth considering if you are manufacturing problems in order to continue avoiding an uncomfortable situation. How do you know the difference? One determining factor might be if you have been through numerous counselors and find that you react negatively to each one. At the same time, it is better to err on the side of going with your gut rather than doubting yourself. You must be able to feel some level of comfort in the beginning, and it may take several sessions to determine if the person is a good fit for you. You are never, ever obligated to continue therapy with someone just because you attended more than one session. There is no contract requiring you to continue when you are not comfortable doing so. If deciding to leave a person, for whatever reason, despite how scary it might be, having a discussion with the therapist about why you believe it is not a good fit may itself be therapeutic and bring about some answers for you.

During the first session, and all early sessions, notice how you feel in the room with the clinician. You probably feel nervous and on edge, worrying at all times what this person thinks of you and if they can be trusted. Take note as to whether you feel heard, respected, and valued for your individuality and opinions. Does the therapist appear to have compassion and hope or are they maybe more interested in proving how knowledgeable or "helpful" he or she is? Can the clinician take feedback or acknowledge mistakes? Do you get the feeling that he or she is going to be advising you and telling you what you should or should not be doing, or, instead, might you be encouraged to make your own decisions? In the end, trust your instincts.

Generally, if a person appears rigid, particularly without explanation to their position on a given issue, arrogant, overly emotional, or closed off to your perspective, these are good signs to keep looking. A therapist needs to be able to demonstrate healthy boundaries, an ability to withstand the inevitable emotional chaos that often arises with trauma, and to remain consistently stable. And so, a firm framework that offers predictability (set day/

time, clear agreement on contact between sessions, cancellation policies that are maintained within reason, etc.) and limits are also necessary. Any agreements made up front as to scheduling, finances, and methods of contact should be kept as consistent as best possible. Of course, sometimes life happens and changes need to be made, but this should be rare and done with openness to how it impacts you, the client, rather than inducing an increased sense of disorganization.

If the clinician is engaging in troublesome or concerning behaviors, do not feel that you need to ignore these just because they are an authority figure or so-called expert. Some examples of problematic behaviors that I have personally heard about or witnessed or that were described by participants include: checking one's phone or email during a session; falling asleep; poor hygiene; looking for praise or recognition from you; asking for favors or advice; talking about personal issues that are not related to the discussion at hand; suggesting or agreeing to a dual relationship of some sort; eating during a session (though, maybe this is therapeutic if discussed and agreed upon with client in advance); inappropriate commentary on the way one looks or how one dresses; and initiating physical contact, such as a hug. Though there are always exceptions and nothing is absolute, these behaviors are generally not okay.

If you find yourself feeling like you have to lie or withhold information, ask yourself why? Do you feel that your therapist will only approve of you if you agree with him or her? Take a chance and be honest and/or disagree—what happens? If your therapist gets upset or shames you, this is a major red flag.

It is also important to work with someone who has been in his or her own therapy. This is a completely appropriate question to ask, and if the clinician treats it otherwise then keep looking. For someone to work in the position of a therapist, they *must* have had some experience with the process themselves and have done work on their own self. You want to be able to work with someone who has some transparency and is not afraid to be a real person with you. A clinician who thinks they can enter into such a delicate relationship with a vulnerable person without having worked through his or her own issues can be dangerous. This is the most likely person to have problems with boundaries, judgments, panicked reactivity to stories of trauma or self-harm/voices/suicidality/and so on, or acting out their own past within the therapeutic relationship. Though risking being extreme, I feel confident in suggesting that one should never engage in therapy with a person who has not themselves been in therapy.

Perhaps most importantly, you should feel a sense of hope that this person might be able to *help* and *support* you, not fix you (because you do not need to be fixed and no one can "fix" someone else anyway). In the first session, consider if the clinician is focused on what is wrong with you or, instead, what happened to you. Having someone tell you what is wrong with you and all the ways that you need to be fixed might feel comforting initially, and also will likely resonate with your internal sense of defectiveness. Yet, this rarely results in true long-term change or healing. Similarly, guarantees and definitive answers are comforting; they also should be considered as warning signs. Therapy, especially after years of chronic adversity and/or trauma, is a long process with few short-term gains. Working through the complex layers of adaptations, hurts, fears, and belief systems is an art form without certainty and can take years to navigate through. While hope is essential, guarantees are an illusion.

Despite the long-term process, therapists should also be able to offer short-term tools or referrals to specialists that can help alleviate acute distress, such as panic, sleep problems, despair, rage, and intense fear. Sometimes, psychiatric drugs may be a helpful tool in this regard; however, anyone who insists this is *necessary* or is a good long-term solution needs to be approached with caution. Patience is paramount, and the only way to withstand this process is to feel comfortable in a safe, respectful, healthy, collaborative relationship where extreme emotions are tolerated and curiosity abounds.

Where to find a therapist:

- Ask friends, family, general practitioners, teachers, or other known acquaintances who have had a positive experience with their therapist or maybe know someone who has. Note that the clinician's educational degree is largely irrelevant, with the exception that psychiatrists (medical doctors, MDs) usually only prescribe and do not do therapy. Otherwise, when it comes to therapists, degree does not matter nearly as much as experience and personality.
- Professional organizations, most of which have an online "find-a-therapist" function, that may offer a trauma-informed approach:

  - International Society for Psychological and Social Approaches to Psychosis
  - International Society for Ethical Psychiatry and Psychology
  - International Society for the Study of Trauma and Dissociation
  - International Society for Traumatic Stress Studies
  - Psychology Today

- Training clinics—While there is a greater chance that these clinics are based on a medical-model, drug-based paradigm, working with an intern or other trainee can be a great way to get low- to no-fee services. Trainees are under supervision of an experienced clinician who generally is monitoring the trainee consistently and ensuring that quality care is being provided. Further, good supervision usually involves challenging the trainee to evaluate his or her own reactions, forcing an exploration of confusing dynamics or problems that may arise in the therapeutic relationship, and providing a sense of safety and support for the trainee so that he or she, in turn, can provide this for the client. Of course, rules tend to be much more rigid, trainees are often trying to prove themselves and so may be too tied to theory or protocol at the expense of listening or attunement, and such relationships rarely last more than one year before the trainee moves on to the next position. Nonetheless, this is a low-cost alternative for some and may offer many useful opportunities.
- Your insurance company—This is the most convoluted and difficult option for searching for a clinician, yet may be the only option when needing to ensure you are covered. Though time-consuming and tedious, sifting through the vast network offered by your insurance company may yield excellent results. If your insurance company does not offer many choices, however, or you do not find a good fit through this network, seek other options. Sometimes no care is better than settling for whatever your insurance company dictates.

Questions to ask a potential therapist:

- How long have you been practicing?
- What is your training?
- Have you ever been in therapy?
- What is your perspective on diagnoses?
- Have you worked with people who have similar experiences to my own? What experience do you have working with [my complaints]?
- Describe what a typical therapy session might look like.
- What is your opinion of collaboration?

Resources

A lot of online things are very safe because you're not in the space with the person and you can close the laptop. And, you can make a lot of choices without explaining them or defending them, which is very safe. P4

The Facebook groups are really helpful. Just, some really awesome friends that I've made online, who, if I'm having a really tough time I can, ya know, talk to them, and I know who's going to be able to calm me down. P6

I've found online support groups or online forum groups to be helpful. Because they are for a broader [population], it's a source of support where people are, I guess, in the same, share a lot of the same experiences and are also therapists in their own way. There's also just respect and freedom to seek out other resources and seek out understanding and, yeah, it's like a comfortable place to go back to. P7

Formal peer support, in clinics or otherwise, continues to accumulate evidence for the healing opportunities they provide (see Chap. 9). Additionally, utilizing the vast network on the internet can be a great way to find support, ideas, and comradery without ever having to leave one's home. It provides a chance to remain anonymous, low commitment, and a safe way to explore oneself without shame. At the same time, one can become overwhelmed looking through the infinite perspectives and conflicting ideas regarding particular phenomena; one must proceed with caution and stick with what resonates, personally, for you.

There are many websites dedicated to the topic of mental health, where active conversations and forums exist. Videos of people speaking about their experiences also abound across cyberspace. Moreover, there are specific online sites that offer free downloads and handouts providing education, general information, coping tools, inspiration, and so on. In addition to spaces focused on mental health issues, it also can be helpful to broaden the search and seek out more spiritually based or existential type resources focused on finding purpose, making meaning, and self-discovery.

Connecting with others via the internet and/or exploring ideas and trying to make meaning using online resources can be an important part of the journey. At the same time, there does lack intimacy, and it cannot replace real, in-person interactions with others. Many of the resources found online can themselves be a portal to finding groups or like-minded individuals in the real world. The following suggested groups and/or organizations can be found online and may or may not also offer information about finding resources in person—this is by no means an all-encompassing list, but rather a starting point that some might find useful.

Peer-Led Initiatives

- Hearing Voices Network (www.hearing-voices.org)—HVN is an international collaboration between professionals, people with lived experience, and their families to develop an alternative approach to coping with emotional distress that is empowering and useful to people, and does not start from the assumption that they have a chronic illness.
- The Voice Collective (www.voicecollective.co.uk)—Offers an online support forum for children and young people who hear voices, see visions, have other "unusual" sensory experiences or beliefs. They also offer support for parents/families and training for youth workers, social workers, mental health professionals, and other supporters.
- Inner Compass Initiative (www.theinnercompass.org)—The resources on the ICI and The Withdrawal Project websites include a detailed layperson's "Companion Guide" to safer tapering from psychiatric medications; mini-booklets that provide detailed, critical information about psychiatric drugs, psychiatric diagnoses, and the mental health industry; and two networking platforms to help people who are thinking critically about the mental health system or seeking support for psychiatric drug withdrawal to find each other in their local communities.
- The Dissociative Initiative (https://di.org.au)—For, by, and about people with multiplicity, dissociation, and amnesia.
- The Icarus Project (theicarusproject.net)—The Icarus Project is a support network and education project by and for people who experience the world in ways that are often diagnosed as mental illness.

In addition to online resources, there are numerous books and other reading materials that may offer guidance, education, and/or theoretical ideas that many might find beneficial. Often, reading stories of others' journeys and experiences can help a person feel less alone and even understood. Books, blogs, articles, and memoirs can also be a great way for a person to explore different ways of making sense of one's own experiences and discover for his or her self what makes most sense, without feeling obliged to agree with someone one knows personally (like a therapist). The following suggested readings are only a starting point and, of course, biased by my own ideas of what makes sense. They also are in addition to the numerous references that can be found throughout this book. Find for yourself what calls to you.

Suggested Readings

- *Living with Voices: 50 Stories of Recovery* by Marius Romme, Sandra Escher, and Jacque Dillon
- *Lucky* by Alice Sebold
- *Agnes's Jacket* by Gail Hornstein
- *The Body Keeps the Score* by Bessel van der Kolk
- *Blind to Betrayal* by Jennifer Freyd and Pamela Birrell
- *The Divided Self* by R. D. Laing
- *Rethinking Madness* by Paris Williams
- *A Fight to Be* by Ron Bassman
- *Mad in America* by Robert Whitaker
- *Pseudoscience in Biological Psychiatry* by Colin Ross and Alvin Pam
- *Deadly Medicines and Organized Crime: How Big Pharma has Corrupted Healthcare* by Peter Gøtzsche
- *Recovery Is My Best Revenge* by Carolyn Spring
- *When the Body Says No* by Gabor Maté
- *Alternatives Beyond Psychiatry* by Peter Stastny and Peter Lehmann

TIPS AND TRICKS

Journals are a good idea. P2

Talking out loud to the different alters I have has been really helpful. P3

I try to take care of my physical body too, as much as I'm able, 'cause it helps me feel better about myself and if I feel better, ya know, physically, that's very helpful with my emotional and my mental health too, I've found. P6

I mean I've meditated since before I even knew what it was, really. But, I try and weave the concepts into my daily living. So, when I'm feeling a bit out of it, I'll try and feel the texture of the couch and I'll actually get to know it like I'm a baby. P8

Sensory things, when I'm dissociating, just different sensory things. Snow has been the biggest one for me to ground. Another grounding one I was taught was to pick out 10 things that are purple cause I have to turn my head—I will get just tunnel vision and only stare forward when I'm dissociating. P9

I guess just stuff I enjoy. Like I have a messy fish tank and keeping that going. And, [keeping] plants healthy and stuff, that's distracting and fun to do and it's nice to look at. P11

> For anxiety—this is a calm ball. It's the most bouncy ball you will ever come across in your entire life. It's designed for big dogs. But, it's solid rubber and you can get it at a pet store ... it really did help with anxiety. P12

Having a tool chest full of different tricks to pull out in times of need is important for all of us. Engaging in regular exercise, maintaining healthy eating habits, getting regular sleep, and finding joyful activities (i.e., having fun!) are part of an overall healthy lifestyle that allows for growth and healing to occur. These are just some of the basics. In addition to fundamental healthy lifestyle choices, however, there are many specific suggestions from participants and others with lived experience that may be helpful.

In general, having a routine and structure allows a person to feel safe and offers some amount of predictability and stability. Having a regular routine also allows for scheduling in self-care activities and gaining better awareness of when distress might be triggered or increased. If you know that, for instance, the evenings tend to be the worst time, then you can plan activities in the evening that will be relaxing, engaging, and/or distracting as a preemptive measure.

At times when anxiety, sadness, fear, voices, dissociation, panic, and/or flashbacks become acutely intense, the best thing to do is not to react with more panic or anger. These are the times to be most gentle with yourself and react with care and compassion. Keep breathing and begin using some tools. It can be helpful to have some of the most useful tricks written down somewhere that can quickly and easily be accessed, like a small, laminated card kept in your pocket. This is also the best time to reach out for support, whether it be to a therapist or peer support, or simply just saying "hi" to an acquaintance. Connecting with another human being in any way can be extremely helpful in grounding you in the present and decreasing the intensity of these painful experiences.

Coping with voices/alters/negative beliefs can be difficult, but there are some ways to combat the overall distress. Talking aloud to these voices and negotiating with them can be a helpful way to challenge harmful and abusive things being said. Try to not believe the hurtful things they say and use selective listening (rather than ignoring) to choose what to take away from what they say. Distraction can also be helpful when they are too powerful, as is engaging in some kind of soothing activity, such as taking a bath or playing relaxing music.

Using sensory tools can also be powerful, especially when feeling trapped in anxiety or dissociation. This means stimulating your senses in some way that forces your brain to focus. Some ways you can do this include: changing your physical position, standing up, balancing on one foot, touching a rough or soft surface or object, squeezing a ball, holding an ice cube, taking a cold shower, snapping a rubber band on your wrist, sucking on a hard candy, drinking tea, describing aloud and in very specific detail some object in your sight, listening to music, rubbing your feet along the floor, smelling incense or oils, and wrapping yourself in a soft blanket.

The following is a list of specific tools that individuals have found to be helpful at different times and for different things. Try and discover what works for you, and be creative!

- Journaling
- Breath work
- Meditation
- Exercise
- Listening to or making music
- Enjoying or creating art
- Watching or engaging in theater
- Improv comedy
- Watching television or movies
- Reading
- Helping others
- Engaging in spiritual activities
- Cooking
- Learning a new skill or formal education
- Touching soft objects
- Holding a stuffed animal
- Going for a walk
- Having a pet
- Playing a sport
- Imagery or visualization of positive narratives
- Drawing on oneself instead of self-harm
- Teaching others
- Finding a hobby
- Fidget toys
- Bouncing a ball

- Stimulating one of the five senses: hold an ice cube, take a cold shower, suck on a candy, describe in detail something in your visual space, listen to soothing sounds, aroma therapy
- Engaging in human contact, even if it is just a stranger

At the end of the day, we all are on our own unique journeys of discovery, growth, and healing. What works for one person may not for another, and each of us benefits from a unique combination of experiences in life. We must be free to choose what works best for us, and to trust that innately we do know what we, personally, need to be fulfilled and reach self-actualization. None of us can do it alone though; mental health services is only one of many, many resources out there. At the end of the day, we all need to connect with others, learn to build healthy and intimate relationships, and find love and compassion. Sometimes it really is that simple, and yet that hard.

INDEX[1]

---

[1] Note: Page numbers followed by 'n' refer to notes.

© The Author(s) 2018
N. Hunter, *Trauma and Madness in Mental Health Services*,
https://doi.org/10.1007/978-3-319-91752-8

G
Genetics, 5, 71, 130–134, 136n1,
136n2, 136n3
Grounding techniques, 229
Guild interests, *see* Conflicts of interest

H
Hallucinations
auditory (*see* Voice-hearing)
sensory/somatic, 8, 30, 31, 34
visual, 34
Hallucinogens, 109
Hearing Voices Network (HVM), 172,
211, 212, 228
Heritability, 131, 132
Hospitalization, 11, 13, 58n7, 169,
170, 183, 191–193
Hypnosis
controversies of, 173
historical, 26
modern use of, 26, 28
Hysteria
comparison with DSM diagnoses, 25
treatment of, 25, 26, 33
Hysterical psychosis, 29, 31

I
Ideology, 8, 15, 35, 46, 50, 52–57,
58n7, 78, 79, 83n1, 102, 106,
127, 134, 135, 136n1, 136n2, 193
Insel, Thomas, 55
Insight, 6, 55, 75, 107, 151, 157,
171, 191, 192, 208, 212
See also Anosognosia
Integration, 9, 159, 171, 173
Internal Family Systems (IFS), 13,
104–105, 153, 170–171
Involuntary commitment, 190
See also Force

J
Janet, Pierre, 4, 24–29, 33, 73, 76,
102, 123, 173
contributions, 4, 24–26, 29,
102, 173
downfall of, 25, 26, 28, 33
Journaling, 168, 231
Jung, Carl, 29, 108, 109

K
Kraepelin, Emil, 29, 31

L
Latent schizophrenia, 5, 6, 10, 11, 13,
15, 18n1, 24, 29–33, 35, 36n3,
36n4, 37n5, 55, 56, 70–77, 80,
84n6, 106–110, 121, 124, 126,
131, 132, 136n3, 155, 157, 160,
173, 184, 187
Lived experience, 9, 12, 17, 160, 169,
183, 206, 207, 211, 228, 230

M
Malleus Maleficarum, 67
Meaning-making, 53, 76, 98, 109,
161, 162, 166, 172, 174n1,
188, 211, 212, 227
Medications, *see* Psychotropic drugs
Memories
accuracy of, 203
direct work with, 82, 159, 204
problems with, 19n2, 203, 204
Mesmer, Franz Anton, 24
Meyer, Adolph, 29
Mindfulness, 13, 77, 109,
134, 210
Multiple personality disorder
(MPD), 6, 24, 33, 34, 99–102

Printed in the United States
By Bookmasters